Children in Intensive Care

*For Mary Pow ... a shining light in life,
and for Andy ... my inspiration,
with love, JD*

*For Martin and Cherry Hassell,
with love, LLH*

For Churchill Livingstone:

Senior Commissioning Editor: Ninette Premdas
Project Manager: Gail Murray
Project Development Manager: Mairi McCubbin
Designer: George Ajayi

Children in Intensive Care

A Nurse's Survival Guide

Joanna H Davies DipN RGN RSCN ENB 415

Sister,
Paediatric Intensive Care Unit,
Guy's and St Thomas' NHS Trust,
Guy's Hospital, London, UK

Lynda L Hassell DipN RGN RSCN ENB 415

Sister,
Paediatric Intensive Care Unit,
Guy's and St Thomas' NHS Trust,
Guy's Hospital, London, UK

Foreword by

Ian Murdoch FRCP DCH BSc MBBS

Director of Paediatric Intensive Care Unit,
Guy's and St Thomas' NHS Trust,
Guy's Hospital, London, UK

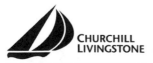
CHURCHILL
LIVINGSTONE

EDINBURGH   LONDON   NEW YORK   PHILADELPHIA   ST LOUIS
SYDNEY   TORONTO   2001

CHURCHILL LIVINGSTONE
An imprint of Harcourt Publishers Limited

© Harcourt Publishers Limited 2001

📙 is a registered trademark of Harcourt Publishers Limited

The right of Joanna Davies and Lynda Hassell to be identified
as authors of this work has been asserted by them in
accordance with the Copyright, Designs and Patents Act 1988

First published 2001

ISBN 0 443 06178 5

British Library Cataloguing in Publication Data
A catalogue record for this book is available from the
British Library

Library of Congress Cataloging in Publication Data
A catalog record for this book is available from the
Library of Congress

Note
Medical knowledge is constantly changing. As new
information becomes available, changes in treatment,
procedures, equipment and the use of drugs become
necessary. The authors and the publishers have taken care to
ensure that the information given in this text is accurate and
up to date. However, readers are strongly advised to confirm
that the information, especially with regard to drug usage,
complies with the latest legislation and standards of practice.

The
Publisher's
policy is to use
paper manufactured
from sustainable fores

Printed in China

Contents

Foreword

Children's intensive care has developed rapidly over the last ten years. In the UK, it has grown from a haphazardly organised service, where children were managed by a variety of physicians with differing specialist backgrounds, into a service managed in the majority by physicians trained specifically in paediatric intensive care.

Likewise, children's intensive care nursing has developed rapidly. Where the late 1980s saw the development of the ENB 415 (Intensive Care Nursing of Children) course, the 1990s saw a rapid expansion of programmes leading to a BSc in Nursing with children's critical care as the focus. Where the ENB 415 course was seen as the gold standard in nurse education, it is now seen as the foundation for developing education to degree level. Postgraduate courses are also available for those nurses wishing to develop advanced nursing skills in clinical practice.

This quick reference pocket book will enable professionals in many settings to access current information, which can only benefit the critically ill child. The knowledge required to work with critically ill children ranges from detailed anatomy and physiology, and pathophysiology, to social and psychological issues. In PICUs, the boundaries between medical and nursing practice are often blurred, with experienced nurses teaching and supporting junior doctors at the bedside. In some settings, healthcare professionals may not encounter critically ill children on a regular basis. This book provides a quick reference resource for medical, nursing and paramedical staff in all settings, enabling them to access information quickly, on a variety of subjects.

The range of topics covered provides information from initial resuscitation and airway management to ongoing treatment of critically ill children with multiple problems. The layout ensures that details are easily accessible, in the form of lists, tables and diagrams. The information given focuses specifically on infants and children and, therefore, provides a useful guide, particularly where local guidelines are not currently available. As stated by the authors, however, it is important to use this information in the context of local guidelines when these are available, particularly when referring to drug dosages.

Ian Murdoch

Preface

The concept of this book began in the notepads of paediatric intensive care nurses, who care for critically ill children with a huge variety of conditions including complex cardiac defects, bronchiolitis, meningococcal septicaemia and specific metabolic disorders. It was evident that a quick point of reference was required which outlined handy hints for emergency situations, and gave practical tips for coping with acutely ill children and troubleshooting technical equipment, together with normal values and drug equations. This is not intended as a textbook but aims to complement such books by providing instant access to concise, valuable nuggets of information, which we hope will stimulate a desire to seek out more in-depth knowledge.

This quick-reference guide is intended for all nurses who come into contact with critically ill children, in accident and emergency departments, general paediatric wards, high dependency units, paediatric and adult intensive care units, and theatres. It will be a useful pocket companion.

We have tried to select data that we have found particularly useful on a day-to-day basis and amalgamated it into a portable format. We have endeavoured to provide concise and up-to-date information but, as treatments and drug doses change rapidly, please also consult local policies, paediatric formularies and current research.

Joanna Davies
Lynda Hassell

London 2000

Acknowledgements

The authors wish to thank and acknowledge the help, advice and support from the following people:

Carmen Barton, Clinical Nurse Specialist, Paediatric Renal Team, Guy's Hospital

Paula Childs, Paediatric Triage Nurse Practitioner, Basildon Hospital

Mollie Cook, Family Support Nurse, Guy's Hospital

Frances Court Brown, Senior Paediatric Dietician, Guy's Hospital

Andrew Durward, Consultant Paediatric Intensivist, Guy's Hospital

Judith Harris, Lecturer Practitioner, Guy's Hospital

Caz Holmes, Paediatric Resuscitation Officer, Guy's Hospital

Fiona Lynch, Senior Staff Nurse, PICU, Guy's Hospital

Corinne Marchant, Transplant Co-ordinator, South East Thames

Michael Marsh, Consultant Paediatric Intensivist, Southampton General Hospital

Gavin Morrison, Consultant Paediatric Intensivist, Diana, Princess of Wales Hospital, Birmingham

Ian Murdoch, Consultant Paediatric Intensivist, Guy's Hospital

Stephen Tomlin, Senior Paediatric Pharmacist, Guy's Hospital

Robert Urquhart, Senior Paediatric Pharmacist, The Royal Free Hospital

Edward Koa Wing, Chief Medical Technologist, Guy's Hospital

– and all their colleagues in paediatric intensive care at Guy's Hospital, London.

We particularly wish to thank Carol Williams, Lead Nurse for Children's Critical Care Services, Guy's Hospital, for her continued guidance and support.

Abbreviations

ABC	Airway, breathing, circulation
ABG	Arterial blood gas
ADH	Anti-diuretic hormone
A&E	Accident and Emergency
ALP	Alkaline phosphatase
ALT	Alanine transaminase
APTT	Activated prothrombin time
ARDS	Adult respiratory distress syndrome
ARF	Acute renal failure
ASD	Atrial septal defect
AV node	Atrio-ventricular node
BP	Blood pressure
BPA	British Paediatric Association
bpm	Beats per minute
BSA	Body surface area
cAMP	Cyclic adenosine monophosphate
CBF	Cerebral blood flow
CBV	Cerebral blood volume
CCF	Congestive cardiac failure
CFAM	Cerebral function analysing monitor
CMV	Controlled mandatory ventilation; cytomegalovirus
CNS	Central nervous system
CO	Cardiac output
CO_2	Carbon dioxide
COHb	Carboxyhaemoglobin
CPAP	Continuous positive airways pressure
CPB	Cardiopulmonary bypass
CPDA	Added citrate, phosphate, dextrose and adenine
CPP	Cerebral perfusion pressure
CPR	Cardiopulmonary resuscitation
CSF	Cerebrospinal fluid
CT	Computerised tomography
CVP	Central venous pressure
CVVH	Continuous veno-venous haemofiltration
CVVHD	Continuous veno-venous haemodiafiltration
DDAVP	1-deamino 8-D arginine vasopressin
DGH	District general hospital
DI	Diabetes insipidus
DIC	Disseminated intravascular coagulation
DKA	Diabetic keto-acidosis

DO_2	Oxygen delivery
DOH	Department of Health
DPT	Diptheria/tetanus/polio vaccine
ECG	Electrocardiogram
ECMO	Extracorporeal membrane oxygenation
EEG	Electroencephalogram
EMD	Electromechanical dissociation
ESR	Erythrocyte sedimentation rate
ET	Endotracheal
ETT	Endotracheal tube
EVD	External ventricular drain
FBC	Full blood count
FFP	Fresh frozen plasma
FiO_2	Fractional concentration of inspired oxygen
FRC	Functional residual capacity
GGT	Gamma-glutamyl transpeptidase
H^+	Hydrogen ion
Hb	Haemoglobin
HCO_3	Carbonic acid
HFO	High-frequency oscillation
HFOV	High-frequency oscillation ventilation
Hib	*Haemophilus influenzae*
ICP	Intracranial pressure
INR	International normalised ratio
IO	Intraosseous
IT	Inspired time
IV	Intravenous
JET	Junctional ectopic tachycardia
kPa	Kilopascal
LDH	Lactate dehydrogenase
LFT	Liver function tests
MAP	Mean airways pressure; mean arterial pressure
MCH	Mean corpuscular haemoglobin
MCS	Microscopy, culture and sensitivity
MCV	Mean corpuscular volume
MRI	Magnetic resonance imaging
$NaHCO_3$	Sodium bicarbonate
NO	Nitric oxide
NO_2	Nitrogen dioxide
O_2	Oxygen
OH^-	Hydroxyl ion
P_aCO_2	Partial pressure of carbon dioxide in arterial blood
P_aO_2	Partial pressure of oxygen in arterial blood
PAP	Pulmonary arterial pressure
PC	Pressure control
PCV	Packed cell volume
PD	Peritoneal dialysis

PDA	Patent ductus arteriosus
PEA	Pulseless electrical activity
PEEP	Positive end-expiratory pressure
PICU	Paediatric intensive care unit
PIP	Peak inspiratory pressure
PPT	Partial prothromboplastin time
PRT	Paediatric retrieval team
PRVC	Pressure-regulated volume control
PS	Pressure support
PT	Prothrombin team
PTV	Patient trigger ventilation
RBC	Red blood cells
RSV	Respiratory syncytial virus
SA node	Sino-atrial node
SAGM	Added sodium chloride, adenine, glucose and mannitol
SaO_2	Oxygen saturation
SIADH	Syndrome of inappropriate antidiuretic hormone secretion
SIMV	Synchronised intermittent mandatory ventilation
SVT	Supraventricular tachycardia
TOF	Tetralogy of Fallot
TPN	Total parenteral nutrition
UKCC	United Kingdom Central Council
VC	Volume control
VF	Ventricular fibrillation
VS	Volume support
VSD	Ventricular septal defect
VT	Ventricular tachycardia
WBC	White blood cell
WPW	Wolf–Parkinson–White syndrome

ALL ABOUT RESUSCITATION

Recognition and prompt treatment of cardiorespiratory deterioration in children is a vital aspect of paediatric nursing in any environment but is particularly pertinent to paediatric intensive care. The ABC method of assessment can be used and children should be frequently reassessed as their condition may rapidly alter.

CARDIOPULMONARY ASSESSMENT

A Airway
B Breathing
C Circulation.

Airway

- Assess patency
- Assess ability to maintain independently with positioning and suction, or
- Assess need for adjuncts, e.g. rigid airway or endotracheal tube.

Breathing

Assess rate of breathing, depth, chest movement, air entry, the work of breathing, use of accessory muscles, recession, nasal flaring, grunting, wheeze, stridor, colour of patient.

Circulation

- Assess heart rate, blood pressure, central and peripheral pulses, skin perfusion, colour, mottling, capillary refill time, temperature – central and peripheral.

See Table 1.5 (p. 14) for normal ranges of heart rate, blood pressure and respiratory rates for each age group.

A quick guide for normal systolic blood pressure in a child 1 year or above

Median systolic blood pressure in children over 1 year of age: 90 mmHg + (2 × age in years)

Pulse volume is related to pulse pressure, i.e. the difference between the systolic and diastolic pressure. When there is decreased cardiac output, the pulse pressure narrows and pulses become weak.

It is also helpful to note level of consciousness, position, pupil reaction, muscle tone, urine output.

SHOCK

This is defined as inadequate delivery of oxygen and metabolic substrates to meet the metabolic demands of the tissues, which results in inadequate organ and tissue perfusion. This in turn can lead to anaerobic metabolism, lactic acidosis, multisystem organ failure and death.

Usually, shock is associated with low cardiac output, but in early septic shock there may be a high-output state with bounding pulses. At this stage there is low systemic vascular resistance and increased blood flow to the skin but there may be a mismatch in distribution of blood flow to the tissues. This can result in tissue hypoxia and eventually a lactic acidosis.

In shock with a low cardiac output there is an increased sympathetic drive, raising the systemic vascular resistance, maintaining the blood pressure and hence perfusion. This diverts blood flow away from non-essential areas, e.g. skin and gut, to increase flow to essential areas, e.g. brain and heart. Clinically a patient in this state will appear pale, feel cool to the touch and have poor peripheral perfusion (American Heart Association 1997).

Shock may be:

- hypovolaemic
- cardiogenic
- septic
- neurogenic
- anaphylactic.

A child in shock will require cardiovascular support with fluid resuscitation and/or inotropic support.

It is useful to classify shock as either compensated or decompensated.

Compensated shock

($\downarrow$ cardiac output, normal blood pressure and $\uparrow$ systemic vascular resistance index.)

The child will have a tachycardia and signs of poor peripheral perfusion, e.g. increased capillary refill time, but will have a normal blood pressure at this stage. The child may have a normal level of consciousness but some signs of inadequate tissue perfusion may become apparent, e.g. increasing lactic acidosis.

Table 1.1   Classification of haemorrhagic shock: the effect on five systems (modified from American College of Surgeons 1989 and as cited in Hazinski 1992 Fleischer G R, Ludwig S 1988 Textbook of Pediatric Emergency Medicine, 2nd edn. © Lippincott Williams & Wilkins, reproduced with permission)

Degree of shock	I: Very mild – haemorrhage, <15% blood volume loss	II: Mild – haemorrhage, 15–25% blood volume loss	III: Moderate – haemorrhage, 26–39% blood volume loss	IV: Severe – haemorrhage, >40% blood volume loss
Cardiovascular	Heart rate normal or mildly raised, normal pulses, normal blood pressure	Tachycardia, peripheral pulses may be diminished, normal blood pressure	Significant tachycardia, thready peripheral pulses, hypotension	Severe tachycardia, thready central pulses, significant hypotension
Respiratory	Normal pH, rate normal	Normal pH, tachypnoea	Metabolic acidosis, moderate tachypnoea	Significant acidosis, severe tachypnoea
Central nervous system	Slightly anxious	Irritable, confused, combative	Irritable or lethargic, diminished pain response	Lethargic, coma
Skin	Warm, pink, capillary refill time brisk (< 2 s)	Cool extremities, mottling, delayed capillary refill time (> 2 s)	Cool extremities, mottling or pallor, prolonged capillary refill time	Cool extremities, pallor or cyanosis
Kidneys	Normal urine output	Oliguria, increased specific gravity	Oliguria, increased urea	Anuria

Decompensated shock

(↓ cardiac output, ↓ blood pressure as ↑ systemic vascular resistance index no longer able to compensate.)

The child will now be hypotensive with weak or absent central pulses and will have an increasing metabolic acidosis, increased capillary refill, a decreased urine output and an altered level of consciousness, reflective of poor end-organ perfusion. This child will need immediate resuscitation as cardiopulmonary arrest will occur if no treatment is given.

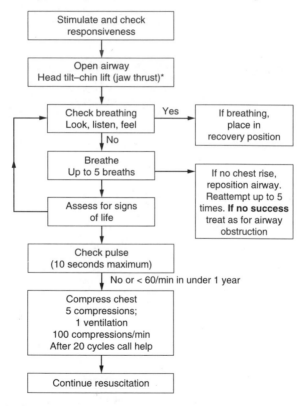

*NB Avoid head tilt if trauma to the neck is suspected; use the jaw thrust to open the airway

Fig. 1.1 Paediatric basic life support algorithm (reproduced with permission from Resuscitation Council (UK) 1998)

Management of shock

- 100% oxygen
- Assess airway and breathing, using adjuncts as necessary
- Establish vascular access – intravenous or intraosseous if necessary
- Use volume expanders and inotropic drugs as required
- Monitor closely.

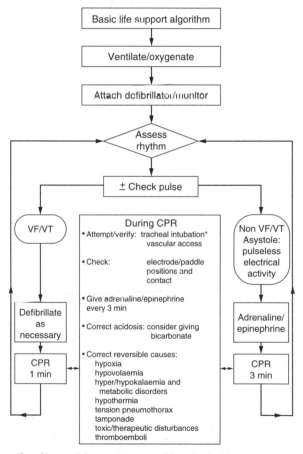

*See Chapter 2 for step-by-step guide to intubation

Fig. 1.2   Paediatric advanced life support algorithm (reproduced with permission from Resuscitation Council (UK) 1998)

Resuscitation drug doses – cardiac arrest (Guy's, St Thomas' and Lewisham Hospitals 1999)

- Epinephrine: initially   10 μg/kg (0.1 mL/kg of 1 in 10 000)
-   then   100 μg/kg (0.1 mL/kg of 1 in 1000)
- Atropine: 15–30 μg/kg

Minimum dose of atropine is 100 μg – to produce vagolytic effects and avoid paradoxical bradycardia (American Heart Association 1997)

- Calcium chloride 10%:   0.1–0.2 mL/kg
- Sodium bicarbonate 8.4%:   1 mL/kg
- Lidocaine 1%:   0.1 mL/kg
- Naloxone: 10 μg/kg
- Isoprenaline: 5 μg/kg
- Adenosine: initially   50 μg/kg
-   then   increase by 50 μg/kg to a maximum dose of 250 μg/kg
- Sodium bicarbonate is used to correct metabolic acidosis. The total number of millimoles of bicarbonate required can be calculated by:

  $F \times$ base deficit (mmol/L) $\times$ weight (kg) where F represents the extracellular fluid : weight ratio.
  - In premature neonates: $F = 0.5\text{-}0.6$
  - In neonates: $F = 0.4$
  - In infants and children: $F = 0.3$.

Only half the base deficit should be corrected initially.

In emergencies it is often difficult to establish intravenous access in infants and children, so consider intraosseous access.

PULSELESS ELECTRICAL ACTIVITY (PEA)

This was previously known as electromechanical dissociation or EMD.

There are recognisable complexes seen on the ECG monitor but there is an absence of palpable pulses and inadequate cardiac output.

Causes of PEA include:

- Severe hypovolaemia (most common cause)
- Severe acidosis
- Severe hypoxaemia ⎫ particularly postoperatively
- Tension pneumothorax ⎭
- Cardiac tamponade
- Profound hypothermia
- Hyperkalaemia
- Drug overdose.

The underlying cause of PEA must be sought but PEA should be treated and managed like asystole until the specific cause has been identified and treated.

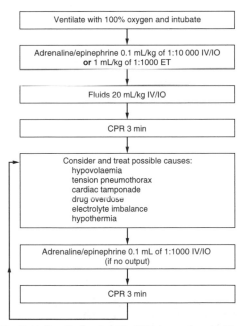

Fig. 1.3 Guidelines for treatment of PEA (reproduced with permission from Guy's, St Thomas' and Lewisham Hospitals 1999)

Table 1.2 Resuscitation schedule; guidelines grouped by age and weight (reproduced with permission from Guy's, St Thomas' and Lewisham Hospitals 1999)

Age	Newborn	6 months	1 year	4 years	8 years
Weight	3 kg	6 kg	10 kg	15 kg	25 kg
Mask	0 or 1	1	1 or 2	1 or 2	3
ET tube	2.5 or 3	3.5 or 4	4 or 4.5	5	6 or 6.5
Fluids/h	12 mL	25 mL	40 mL	50 mL	65 mL
Epinephrine 1:10 000	0.3 mL	0.6 mL	1 mL	1.5 mL	2.5 mL
Epinephrine 1:1000	0.3 mL	0.6 mL	1 mL	1.5 mL	2.5 mL
Atropine	100 µg	120 µg	200 µg	300 µg	500 µg
Ca chloride 10%	0.3 mL	0.6 mL	1 mL	1.5 mL	2.5 mL
Ca gluconate 10%	0.6 mL	1.2 mL	2 mL	3 mL	5 mL
Isoprenaline 200 µg in 10 mL	0.75 mL	1.5 mL	2.5 mL	3.75 mL	6.25 mL
Lidocaine 1%	0.3 mL slowly	0.6 mL slowly	1 mL slowly	1.5 mL slowly	2.5 mL slowly
Sodium bicarbonate 8.4%	–	6 mL	10 mL	15 mL	25 mL
Sodium bicarbonate 4.2%	6 mL slowly	–	–	–	–

Table 1.3 Guidelines for the drug treatment of tachycardia (reproduced with permission from Guy's, St Thomas' and Lewisham Hospitals 1999)

Arrhythmia	Initial treatment
Supraventricular tachycardia	1. Adenosine – repeat bolus when necessary 2. Digoxin 3. Esmolol* 4. Verapamil*
Sinus tachycardia	Find underlying cause
Atrial fibrillation Atrial flutter Atrial tachycardia	1. Digoxin 2. Propranolol 3. Amiodarone
Ventricular tachycardia	1. Lidocaine 2. Amiodarone 3. Magnesium
Wolff–Parkinson–White syndrome with atrial fibrillation	Amiodarone DO NOT GIVE DIGOXIN OR VERAPAMIL

* Refer to specialist information, e.g. Guy's, St Thomas' and Lewisham Hospitals 1999, regarding contraindications of esmolol and verapamil
NB If the patient is compromised then cardioversion is recommended. Expert advice should be sought before the prescription of these drugs.

INTRAOSSEOUS ACCESS

Intraosseous access uses the vascular network in long bones to transport fluids or drugs from the medullary cavity into the circulation.

Sites for intraosseous infusions include the proximal tibia and the medial malleolus.

Advantages of intraosseous access

- Quick, safe and easy to insert
- Medication can be given in the same dose as the intravenous route
- Absorption time has been found to be as effective as intravenous injections in maintaining drug levels.

Contra indications

Not recommended for use:

- on recently fractured bones
- in osteogenesis imperfecta.

  Do not give the drug bretylium via the intraosseous route.

Guidelines on insertion of intraosseous needle in proximal tibia

- Immobilise limb and paint with antiseptic
- Use local anaesthetic down to the periosteum if required, i.e. if patient is conscious
- Use landmarks to assess correct placement
- Palpate tibial tuberosity and grasp the medial aspect of the tibia with the thumb – the optimal site of insertion is halfway between these points and 1–2 cm distal (Spivey 1987)
- The needle is inserted perpendicular to the bone at a 15–30°angle towards the foot, i.e. away from the epiphyseal plate
- Apply downward pressure in a boring motion until a 'pop' is heard and resistance suddenly decreases, indicating that the needle has entered the medullary cavity
- The needle should stand up without support
- Penetration from the skin through the cortex is around 1 cm in an infant or child

- Remove inner stylet, and bone marrow content (like blood) should be aspirated to confirm needle placement
- A transparent dressing may be placed around the entry site
- Medication must be administered under pressure and then flushed well.

Complications include needle clotting, extravasation and rarely infection. If fluid is seen to be entering surrounding tissues, stop the infusion immediately, remove needle and apply pressure to the site. An intraosseous needle can remain in place until other intravascular access is obtained.

USE OF THE DEFIBRILLATOR

The defibrillator can be used both for defibrillation and synchronised cardioversion. All oxygen should be removed from the area before using the defibrillator. Defibrillation pads need to be changed after 6 shocks.

Defibrillation

- is the definitive treatment for ventricular fibrillation (VF) or pulseless ventricular tachycardia (VT) (American Heart Association 1997)
- is the passage of an electrical current through the heart
- is an asynchronised depolarisation of a critical mass of myocardial cells to allow spontaneous reorganised myocardial depolarisation to resume.

Starting dose: 2 J/kg
Subsequent doses: 4 J/kg

 Defibrillation should not be used in asystolic patients: it will not work.

If VF or pulseless VT continue after one defibrillation, the energy level will be increased to 4 J/kg and the second and third defibrillation should be given in rapid succession, pausing in between only to check the rhythm on the monitor. After three shocks have been given CPR and resuscitation drugs should be given before the administration of any further shocks.

Synchronised cardioversion

- is the treatment of choice in patients who have tachy-arrhythmias, e.g. supraventricular tachycardia, ventricular tachycardia with palpable pulses, atrial fibrillation and atrial flutter, who are seen to be cardiovascularly compromised (American Heart Association 1997)
- results in depolarisation of the myocardium but provides depolarisation that is timed with the patient's own intrinsic electrical activity.

 Press the synchroniser mode button on the defibrillator before administering the shock.

Initial dose: 0.5 J/kg
Subsequent dose will be 1 J/kg then 2 J/Kg (APLS Working Group 1997)
The discharge buttons on the paddles must be pressed and held for several QRS complexes when cardioverting.

Choice of paddle

Infant paddles: 4.5 cm, should be used for infants up to 1 year of age or up to 10 kg in weight

Adult paddles: 8–13 cm, should be used in patients older than 1 year of age and more than 10 kg in weight

Defibrillation pads

Defibrillation pads are recommended for use rather than electrode gel or KY jelly.

Electrode paddles should be placed so that the heart is in between them. Anterior to posterior electrode and pad position is superior but difficult. Normally, one pad is placed on the upper right chest below the clavicle and the other to the left of the left nipple in the anterior axillary line.

 A mirror image electrode placement is necessary if the patient has dextrocardia.

USEFUL MNEMONICS

Assessment tool: ABCDEFG
A airway
B breathing
C circulation
D don't
E ever
F forget
G glucose
  – particularly in the fitting child.

Common postresuscitation airway complications: DOPE
D displacement of endotracheal tube
O obstruction of endotracheal tube
P pneumothorax
E equipment failure

Emergency drugs: SCALE
S sodium bicarbonate
C calcium (either chloride or gluconate)
A atropine
L lidocaine (lignocaine)
E epinephrine (adrenaline)

Drugs that can be given via endotracheal tube: LEAN
L lidocaine
E epinephrine
A atropine
N naloxone

Quick assessment tool measuring responsiveness: AVPU (American Heart Association 1997)
A awake
V voice
P pain
U unresponsive

NEWBORN RESUSCITATION

Paediatric intensive care nurses are not often required to resuscitate newborn infants but do need to know the principles if required to do so. Figure 1.4 lists resuscitative procedures in stages: every infant will require stage I but few will need to proceed to stage V. Remember: Airway, Breathing, Circulation.

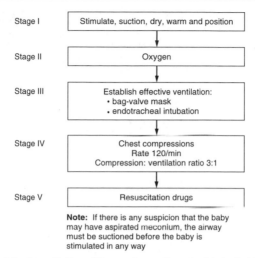

Stage I	Stimulate, suction, dry, warm and position
Stage II	Oxygen
Stage III	Establish effective ventilation: • bag-valve mask • endotracheal intubation
Stage IV	Chest compressions Rate 120/min Compression: ventilation ratio 3:1
Stage V	Resuscitation drugs

Note: If there is any suspicion that the baby may have aspirated meconium, the airway must be suctioned before the baby is stimulated in any way

Fig. 1.4 Resuscitation of the newborn – flow chart (adapted from American Heart Association 1997)

The Apgar score

The Apgar score was developed to indicate a baby's condition at 1 and 5 minutes after birth. Resuscitation should not be delayed while scores are calculated but some knowledge of the scoring system is useful. The maximum score is 10 for a pink, responsive baby who has normal heart rate and respiratory rate, and the minimum score is 0 for a totally unresponsive baby who has no cardiorespiratory function. A score is given to each of five categories as seen in Table 1.4.

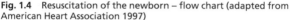

	Table 1.4 Apgar score (adapted with permission from Hull & Johnston 1996)				
Score	**Heart rate**	**Respirations**	**Muscle tone**	**Response to stimulation**	**Colour**
0	Absent	Absent	Flaccid	None	White/blue
1	Slow <100/min	Gasping/ irregular	Some flexion	Facial grimace	Pink body, blue extremities
2	>100/min	Good/ regular	Active movements	Cry/cough	Completely pink

Table 1.5 Normal vital signs – normal values of heart rate, blood pressure and respiratory rate (adapted from Hazinski 1992)

Age of baby/child	Heart rate (beats/min)	Blood pressure (mmHg) Systolic	Diastolic	Respiratory rate (breaths/min)
Newborn (3 kg)	100–180	50– 70	25–45	30–60
Infant	100–160	85–105	55–65	30–60
Toddler	80–110	95–105	55–65	24–40
Preschool	70–110	95–110	55–65	22–34
School age	65–110	95–110	55–70	18–30
Adolescent	60– 90	110–130	65–80	12–16

REFERENCES

Advanced Life Support Group 1997 Advanced paediatric life support. The practical approach, 2nd edn. BMJ Publishing Group, London

American College of Surgeons 1989 Advanced trauma life support course. American College of Surgeons, Chicago, IL

American Heart Association 1997 Pediatric advanced life support, 3rd edn. American Heart Association, Dallas, TX

Fleisher G R, Ludwig S 1988 Textbook of pediatric emergency medicine, 2nd edn. Williams & Wilkins, Baltimore, MD

Guy's, St Thomas' and Lewisham Hospitals 1999 Paediatric formulary, 5th edn. Guy's, St Thomas' and Lewisham Hospitals, London

Hazinski M F (ed) 1992 Nursing care of the critically ill child, 2nd edn. Mosby Year Book, St Louis, MO

Hull D, Johnston D I 1996 Essential paediatrics, 3rd edn. Churchill Livingstone, Edinburgh

Resuscitation Council (UK) 1998 The 1998 resuscitation guidelines for use in the United Kingdom. Resuscitation Council (UK), London

Spivey W H 1987 Intra osseous infusions. J Pediat 111: 639–643

FURTHER READING

British Medical Journal 1993 Advanced paediatric life support. British Medical Journal, London

Blumer J L 1990 A practical guide to pediatric intensive care, 3rd edn. C V Mosby, St Louis, MO

Miccolo M A 1990 Intraosseous infusion. Crit Care Nurse 10(10): 35–47

Versmold H 1981 Aortic blood pressure during the first 12 hours of life in infants with birthweight 610–4220 g. Pediatrics 67–107

AIRWAY, ACID BASE AND VENTILATION

2

In children it is respiratory failure as opposed to cardiac failure that is often the primary reason for resuscitation. Early recognition and treatment may prevent full cardiopulmonary arrest. Knowledge of the anatomy of the respiratory system in infants and children clarifies the reasons why this occurs.

ANATOMY OF THE PAEDIATRIC RESPIRATORY SYSTEM

- Large head, short neck with cartilaginous tracheal rings, which can collapse, causing airway obstruction
- Face and mandible small and hypoplastic in infants
- Relatively large tongue and maybe loose teeth
- The anterior commissure of the glottis is directed caudally and the infant trachea is angled posteriorly, which may hamper the easy passage of the endotracheal tube
- Larynx is high and anterior (at level of 2nd and 3rd cervical vertebrae in infants compared with 5th and 6th vertebrae in adults)
- Cricoid ring is the narrowest part of the airway as opposed to the larynx in adults
- Compliant rib cage, which can lead to inefficiency in inspiration resulting in increased work of breathing
- Poorly developed intercostal muscles with few type 1 fatigue-resistant fibres, which increases the likelihood of respiratory failure secondary to fatigue
- Protuberant abdomen with caudally displaced diaphragm, which impedes efficient contraction.

Some infants are obligate nose-breathers. The ability to breathe orally appears to be acquired between 31 and 34 weeks postconception when the baby also acquires the ability to coordinate sucking and swallowing, but Miller et al (1985) found that only 78% of term babies could sustain oral breathing in response to nasal occlusion. They have narrow nasal passages, which are easily obstructed by mucus. Preterm infants have been found to have increased airway resistance and interrupted periods of oral airway obstruction when they breathe orally (Miller et al 1986).

In children aged 3–8 years, adenotonsillar hypertrophy is a common problem, which tends to cause obstruction, and there may be difficulty when the nasal route is used to pass tracheal or gastric tubes.

Box 2.1   Normal respiratory rates

< 1 year: 30–40 breaths/min
2–5 years: 20–30 breaths/min
5–12 years: 15–20 breaths/min
> 12 years: 12–16 breaths/min

At rest, tachypnoea indicates that increased ventilation is needed because of either lung or airway disease or metabolic acidosis.

Oxygenation

This can be assessed by looking at the child's lip or nail colour but can be measured using pulse oximetry or blood gas analysis. In a critically ill child it is important to measure:

- haemoglobin concentration (Hb)
- oxygen saturation (Sa_{O_2})
- arterial oxygen content (P_aO_2).

Children may be able to cope with mild hypoxia for a short time by increasing their cardiac output but when they become unable to compensate, cardiorespiratory failure will ensue. The following formulae demonstrate the relationships between haemoglobin, oxygen delivery and cardiac output. Oxygen delivery (D_{O_2}) is the amount of oxygen delivered to the tissues per minute

D_{O_2} = Arterial oxygen content × cardiac output (CO)

Cardiac output = heart rate × stroke volume

Arterial oxygen content ($mLO_2/100\,mL$)
= Hb (g/dL) × 1.34 (mLO_2/gHb) × oxyhaemoglobin saturation + ($0.003 \times P_aO_2$)

Haemoglobin which is 100% saturated contains 1.34 mL of bound oxygen.

Normal arterial oxygen content is 18–20 mL of O_2 per 100 mL blood.

VENTILATION AND DEFINITION OF TERMS

- *Ventilation* is the process of movement of gas between the lungs and the ambient air
- *Tidal volume* is the volume of gas that is inspired and expired in one normal breath ($\cong 6\,\text{mL/kg}$)
- *Minute volume* is the quantity of gas expired by the lungs in one minute; minute volume = tidal volume × frequency
- *Functional residual capacity* is the amount of gas that remains in the lungs after normal expiration
- *The anatomical dead space* (around 30% of each tidal volume) fills the conducting airways and no gas exchange takes place there.

Pulse oximetry

This is a noninvasive, reliable and easy-to-use method of calculating a patient's oxygen saturation. The pulse oximeter consists of a photodetector that is wrapped around a pulsatile tissue bed, i.e. on a finger or toe, or on the ear, and two light-emitting diodes that transmit red and infrared light. Oxygenated and deoxygenated haemoglobin absorb these two lights differently and the haemoglobin saturation (percentage of total haemoglobin oxygenated) is inversely related to the amount of red light absorbed.

The pulse oximeter is thought to be accurate to ± 4% when oxygen saturation is 80% or above but below this figure it tends to over-read and may not detect acute changes and severe hypoxaemia. Inaccurate readings may also occur as a result of poor peripheral perfusion, oedema, hypothermia or jaundice, or with abnormal haemoglobins, e.g. methaemoglobin or carboxyhaemoglobin. A raised bilirubin will cause under-reading of the oxygen saturation as the bilirubin absorbs the light but the presence of carboxyhaemoglobin will lead to an overestimation of saturation of the total haemoglobin of blood. The pulse oximeter is also sensitive to movement and this may interfere with readings (Taylor & Whitwam 1986).

Oxyhaemoglobin dissociation curve

The oxyhaemoglobin dissociation curve (Fig. 2.1) shows the non linear relationship between haemoglobin saturation and the partial pressure of oxygen (P_aO_2). Each molecule of

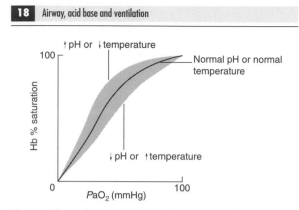

Fig. 2.1 The oxyhaemoglobin dissociation curve, showing the relationship between haemoglobin saturation and pH

haemoglobin is made up of a protein (globin) and a combination of ferrous iron and protophyrin (haem), of which there are four. Each haem group has a different affinity to oxygen. Looking at the oxyhaemoglobin dissociation curve, the first haem group binds moderately easily with oxygen and there is a gentle curve. The second and third haems have the greatest affinity for oxygen and there is a steep slope as the haemoglobin saturation rises with a relatively small change in the P_aO_2. The fourth haem has the greatest difficulty binding to oxygen and so the curve flattens out, relatively less oxygen being taken up per unit change in P_aO_2 as the haemoglobin is reaching near-total saturation, i.e. 97–100%. This occurs when P_aO_2 reaches around 13.3 kPa; there is therefore no additional benefit in keeping a patient's P_aO_2 any higher than this.

If the curve is shifted to the right, then haemoglobin binds less oxygen and is less well saturated at any partial pressure of oxygen. Factors that shift the curve to the right include acidosis, hypercapnia and hyperthermia.

If the curve is shifted to the left, haemoglobin binds more oxygen at any partial pressure of oxygen. Factors that shift the curve to the left include alkalosis, hypocapnia and hypothermia.

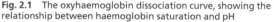

UPPER RESPIRATORY TRACT

Common conditions that affect the upper respiratory tract include croup, epiglottitis, tracheal stenosis or malacia and

Signs of respiratory distress and inadequate ventilation in children

Tachypnoea, cricoid tug, sternal, intercostal or subcostal recession, shoulder rolling, nasal flaring, weak cry, stridor or wheeze, head bobbing, lethargy, decreased responsiveness, irritability, decreased level of consciousness, hypoxaemia, hypercarbia.
Late signs: bradycardia, decreased air movement, apnoea or gasping, poor systemic perfusion.

any respiratory condition that leads to an increase in respiratory secretions.

The airway of infants and children is much smaller than that of adults. Poiseuille's law states:

$$\text{resistance } \alpha \quad \frac{1}{\text{radius}^4}$$

that is, the resistance to airflow is inversely proportional to the fourth power of the radius. In other words, a small amount of mucus in the airway, oedema or tracheal stenosis will significantly increase resistance to airflow and will increase the work of breathing.

A child with upper airway obstruction will be most comfortable sitting up and leaning forwards, may be anxious, restless, cyanosed, tachypnoeic, have an inspiratory stridor, drool, have nasal flaring and be using the accessory muscles to breathe.

LOWER RESPIRATORY TRACT

Common conditions that affect the lower respiratory tract include bronchiolitis, asthma, pneumonia, foreign body aspiration and respiratory distress syndrome. Bronchospasm, increased mucus production, oedema and inflammation of airway mucosa can lead to diffuse air trapping, decreased air movement, decreased compliance and increased work of breathing. A child with lower respiratory tract disease may have an expiratory wheeze, prolonged expiratory time, be tachypnoeic, cyanotic, use accessory muscles, cough and may have hyperinflated lungs.

ACID–BASE BALANCE AND INTERPRETATION OF BLOOD GASES

pH is a term used to describe the acidity or alkalinity of a solution. The pH scale is based on the number of hydrogen ions, expressed in moles per litre. A pH of 7 indicates a neutral solution, e.g. water, where the concentration of hydrogen (H^+) and hydroxyl (OH^-) ions are equal.

- pH below 7 = an acid solution, which dissociates into H^+ ions (cations) and OH^- ions (anions) with more H^+ ions than OH^- ions.
- pH above 7 = an alkaline solution, which dissociates into OH^- ions and H^+ ions with more OH^- ions than H^+ ions.

Three major mechanisms homeostatically control blood pH:

- buffers
- respiration
- renal excretion.

Normal blood pH = 7.35–7.45.

pH levels of below 6.8 and above 7.8 are typically incompatible with life.

If a solution has a pH of 7, this means that it contains one ten-millionth of a mole of H^+ ions per litre. This number, 0.0000001, is written 10^{-7} in exponential form, but pH is a negative log so this is converted to a positive number 7. A change of 1 on the pH scale represents a tenfold change in H^+ concentration.

Buffers

The most important buffer is the carbonic-acid–bicarbonate buffer system in which carbonic acid (H_2CO_3) is the weak acid and sodium bicarbonate ($NaHCO_3$) is the weak base. In solution dissociation occurs:

H_2CO_3	$\leftrightarrow$	H^+	$+$	HCO_3^-
Carbonic acid		hydrogen		bicarbonate
$NaHCO_3$	$\leftrightarrow$	Na^+	$+$	HCO_3^-
Sodium bicarbonate		sodium		bicarbonate.

If the blood becomes very acidic, the sodium bicarbonate disassociates to buffer the acid, thus increasing concentration of carbonic acid and decreasing sodium bicarbonate, but the net result is an increase in pH (as carbonic acid is weak). If there is a strong base in the blood, i.e. the blood is alkaline, the concentration of sodium bicarbonate increases and carbonic acid is used up as the buffer. Other buffer systems include phosphate, haemoglobin–oxyhaemoglobin and protein buffer systems. The phosphate buffer system works in a similar way to the carbonic acid system in the red blood cells and the kidney tubular fluids. The haemoglobin–oxyhaemoglobin buffer system buffers carbonic acid in the blood, while the protein buffer system works in the body cells and plasma.

Respiration

Respirations regulate the level of carbon dioxide (CO_2) in body fluids:

$$CO_2 + H_2O \leftrightarrow H_2CO_3 \leftrightarrow H^+ + HCO_3^-.$$

The level of PCO_2 in the blood gas will signify whether there is a respiratory component. If the PCO_2 is high, this signifies a respiratory acidosis and if it is low, this signifies a respiratory alkalosis. An increased respiratory rate eliminates CO_2 and less H_2CO_3 and H^+ are formed, increasing pH.

Renal secretion

Kidney tubular secretion helps control the pH of blood. If the pH of blood is acidic, there is increased secretion of H^+, which displaces another cation, usually Na^+, which then diffuses from the urine into the tubule cell where it combines with bicarbonate to form sodium bicarbonate, which then gets absorbed into the blood stream. Thus H^+ is lost from the body and the pH becomes less acidic (Tortora & Anagnostakos 1984).

Interpretation of blood gas analyses

When looking at a blood gas, the first thing to notice is the pH – whether it is acidotic, alkalotic or normal. The next

Table 2.1 Normal arterial blood gas values for neonates and children		
	Normal infant/child values	**Normal neonatal values**
pH	7.35–7.45	7.3–7.4
PCO_2 (kPa)	4.5–6.0 (35–45 mmHg)	4.6–6.0 (35–45 mmHg)
PO_2 (kPa)	10–13 (75–100 mmHg)	7.3–12 (55–90 mmHg)
Bicarbonate (mmol/L)	22–26	18–25
Base (mmol/L)	−2 to +2	−4 to + 4

Table 2.2 Acid–base disturbances (reproduced with permission from Easterbrook 1994)

Acid–base abnormality	Primary disturbance	Effect on pH	Effect on P_{O_2}	Base excess	Compensatory response
Respiratory acidosis	↑P_{CO_2}	↓	↓		↑HCO_3^-
Metabolic acidosis	↓HCO_3^-	↓	N or ↑*	−ve	↓P_{CO_2}
Respiratory alkalosis	↓P_{CO_2}	↑	N or ↑*		↓HCO_3^-
Metabolic alkalosis	↑HCO_3^-	↑	N or ↑*	+ve	↑P_{CO_2}

Compensatory mechanism

consideration is the P_{CO_2}: whether high, low or normal. If the P_{CO_2} is high, then there is a respiratory inadequacy, often causing an acidosis; and if it is low this is due to hyperventilation, which causes a respiratory alkalosis, or it may be a compensatory response. P_{O_2} gives some indication of adequate or inadequate oxygenation, but look at oxygen saturation in conjunction with this. The level of base and standard bicarbonate can also be useful. A low bicarbonate and a base deficit indicates a metabolic acidosis, whereas a high bicarbonate and base excess indicates a metabolic alkalosis.

Three abnormal values in a blood gas represent a compensatory mechanism. Metabolic disturbances are compensated acutely by changes in ventilation and chronically by appropriate renal responses. Respiratory disturbances are compensated by renal tubular secretion of hydrogen.

Box 2.2 Common causes of acidosis and alkalosis

Respiratory acidosis
Any cause of hypoventilation:

- Obstructive airways disease, e.g. asthma
- CNS depression, e.g. head injury, encephalitis
- Neuromuscular disease, e.g. myasthenia gravis, Guillain–Barré syndrome
- Artificial ventilation

Respiratory alkalosis
Any cause of hyperventilation:

- Psychogenic, e.g. hysteria, pain
- Central, e.g. raised intracranial pressure, meningitis
- Pulmonary, e.g. hypoxia, pulmonary embolus or oedema, pneumonia

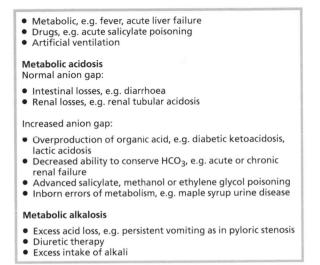

- Metabolic, e.g. fever, acute liver failure
- Drugs, e.g. acute salicylate poisoning
- Artificial ventilation

Metabolic acidosis
Normal anion gap:

- Intestinal losses, e.g. diarrhoea
- Renal losses, e.g. renal tubular acidosis

Increased anion gap:

- Overproduction of organic acid, e.g. diabetic ketoacidosis, lactic acidosis
- Decreased ability to conserve HCO_3, e.g. acute or chronic renal failure
- Advanced salicylate, methanol or ethylene glycol poisoning
- Inborn errors of metabolism, e.g. maple syrup urine disease

Metabolic alkalosis

- Excess acid loss, e.g. persistent vomiting as in pyloric stenosis
- Diuretic therapy
- Excess intake of alkali

In chronic conditions where P_{CO_2} is increased, there is renal compensation and retention of bicarbonate, with pH returning to near normal levels.

Anion gap

It may be useful to calculate the anion gap if the cause of a metabolic acidosis is not known. The anion gap is calculated as the difference between the sum of plasma sodium and potassium and the sum of plasma bicarbonate and chloride concentration:

Anion gap = (sodium + potassium) − (bicarbonate + chloride).

The normal anion gap ranges from 5–12 mmol/L. A patient who has a metabolic acidosis with a normal anion gap will have lost base, e.g. with diarrhoea. A patient with a metabolic acidosis who has an increased anion gap will have gained acid, e.g. in ketoacidosis (Hinds & Watson 1996).

MEANS AND METHODS OF OXYGEN DELIVERY

This can be divided into high- or low-flow methods.

Low flow

Mask, e.g. Venturi – can give wide range of concentrations, i.e. from 35–60% oxygen with a flow rate of 6–10 L/min. The inspired oxygen can only reach 60% as air mixes with oxygen through the exhalation ports in the side of the mask. A minimum flow of 6 L/min must be used to maintain an increased oxygen concentration to prevent rebreathing of exhaled carbon dioxide.

Nasal cannula – a maximum flow rate of 2 L/min is usually prescribed, as higher flow rates will irritate the nasopharynx. However this could vary up to 4 L/min according to manufacturers' instructions.

High flow

Headbox – able to achieve an inspired oxygen concentration of 80–90%. Always use oxygen analyser and titrate oxygen concentration to patient requirement. The flow rate must be 10–15 L/min to prevent accumulation of carbon dioxide (Table 2.3).

Table 2.3 Oxygen concentration versus flow rates	
Oxygen concentration (%)	**Oxygen flow (litres)**
28	4–5
31	6
35	8
40	9
60	10

INDICATIONS FOR ASSISTED VENTILATION

Apnoea, respiratory distress with either increasing P_{CO_2} or decreasing pH and poor oxygenation.

MODES OF VENTILATION

There are many modes of ventilation that can be used on a child requiring ventilatory assistance. One classification distinguishes those with an intact respiratory drive who require minimal help, e.g. pressure support mode or even just continuous positive airways pressure, from others who require more controlled ventilatory support, e.g. in a mandatory ventilation mode. Various modes are explained, highlighting some of the advantages and disadvantages. (Information from 'Pressure-control ventilation' to 'Positive end expiratory pressure (PEEP)' is adapted from Siemens System SV300 1993, with permission.

Pressure-control ventilation

- Used in neonates and infants with poor lung compliance and increased airway resistance
- Flow and pressure are controlled by ventilator settings
- Time cycled: each respiratory cycle is made up by setting the inspired and expired time in seconds
- Continuous flow of gas allowing the infant to interbreathe between ventilator breaths
- Time-triggered ventilator breaths, which may be synchronised or mandatory breaths depending on the ventilator setting
- Volumes are not measured but are dependent on chest compliance and resistance.

The advantage of pressure-controlled ventilation is the avoidance of high airway pressures, but the disadvantage is that there is no guarantee of volume delivered.

Volume-control ventilation

- Used mainly in children over 10 kg
- Tidal volume between 10 and 15 mL/kg
- Preset tidal volume, inspired minute volume, frequency of breaths and inspiratory time
- Pressure is not set but dependent on lung compliance and resistance
- Can be used in many modes.

Controlled mandatory ventilation (CMV)

- Patient receives a preset number of ventilator-generated breaths at a preset tidal volume, at mandatory intervals
- Gas flow is present so that the patient may breathe spontaneously in between each mandatory breath.

Synchronised intermittent mandatory ventilation (SIMV)

- Provides preset breaths at a preset tidal volume, but the breaths are synchronised with the patient's initiation of inspiration. The patient may take additional breaths.

Pressure support (PS)

- Patient initiates a breath, thus generating negative pressure, and then the ventilator provides a breath with preset airways pressure; the amount of negative pressure required to generate a breath is set by altering the trigger sensitivity
- There is no back-up rate
- Patient must generate own rate, inspiratory time and tidal volume.

(Using the Servo ventilators, the trigger is measured in cmH_2O. Thus a trigger of -2 below positive end expiratory pressure (PEEP) requires minimal effort before a breath is delivered but -5 requires more effort. Using the SLE ventilator, the trigger is measured in minimum and maximum sensitivity: therefore, if the trigger is set at 5, this is the most sensitive setting, requiring the least effort to trigger a breath.)

Patient trigger ventilation (PTV)

- Back-up rate is set on the CMV setting using preset inspiratory time, peak inspiratory pressure (PIP) and PEEP to act as a safety mechanism in case of apnoea
- Patient initiates a breath, generates negative pressure and the ventilator will deliver the preset breath at a rate determined by the patient
- Trigger sensitivity must be set to determine the amount of negative pressure required in order that a breath be delivered.

SIMV pressure control and pressure support (SIMV PC & PS)

- Combination of controlled and support ventilation
- Synchronised mandatory breaths at preset rate/min with controlled pressures
- When patient interbreathes and generates a negative pressure, these triggered breaths are pressure-supported (this avoids high airway pressures but the volumes cannot be set).

SIMV volume control and pressure support (SIMV VC & PS)

- Ventilator delivers synchronised mandatory volume-controlled breaths
- When patient makes respiratory effort in between these breaths and generates a negative pressure, these will be pressure supported, i.e. breath is delivered to the preset pressure support set above PEEP.

Pressure-regulated volume control (PRVC)

- Combines the advantages of both pressure and volume control
- Set the tidal and minute volume plus the upper pressure limit
- This mode delivers volumes set with lower inspiratory pressures than in volume control mode.

Volume support (VS)

- Set tidal volumes
- In case of apnoea, preset rate, tidal and minute volumes are set in PRVC and will be delivered and the ventilator will alarm
- Gives lowest inspiratory pressure support to deliver the preset tidal volume
- If lung compliance changes, inspiratory support pressure will be regulated to deliver set tidal volumes.

Continuous positive airways pressure (CPAP)

- Used in patients with intact respiratory drive, as no back-up rate
- Increases or maintains lung volume, opens atelectatic areas of the lungs and can increase functional residual capacity (FRC)
- Patient generates respiratory rate, inspiratory time, tidal volume and peak
- Inspiratory pressure but CPAP maintains a positive end expiratory pressure at all times.

Positive end expiratory pressure (PEEP)

- Increases FRC and maintains lung recruitment
- Improves alveolar ventilation
- Increases arterial oxygen content

- Increases intrathoracic pressure and may impede systemic venous return and thus cardiac output
- High PEEP, i.e. above 8, may impede cerebral venous return, which may increase intercranial pressure.

High-frequency ventilation

This is used in patients who have respiratory failure which has not responded to maximal, conventional ventilation. There are four main types:

- *High-frequency positive pressure ventilation* – conventional ventilation with higher frequencies and smaller tidal volumes
- *High-frequency flow interrupted ventilation* – high frequencies with small tidal volumes and a device to rapidly turn gas flow on and off
- *High-frequency jet ventilation* – gas is delivered through a small bore cannula that extends into the endotracheal or tracheostomy tube, allowing the delivery of large tidal volumes at low airway pressures. There is a device to interrupt flow and to adjust the frequency and inspiratory time. Rates of 30–300 breaths per minute are used
- *High-frequency oscillation ventilation* – uses a continuous gas flow to prevent carbon dioxide accumulation and to provide oxygenation by maintaining recruitment achieved through the application of a constant mean airways pressure while ventilation is achieved at supraphysiological rates around 600 breaths per minute. The tidal volumes are smaller than the anatomical dead space but must exceed the dead space that is machine related (Niederer et al 1994).

Table 2.4 Changes in ventilation and the effect on blood gases (reproduced with permission from Blumer 1990)

	P_aO_2	P_aCO_2
↑ Peak inspiratory pressure	↑	↓
↑ Positive end expiratory pressure	↑	↑
↑ Frequency	↑	↓
↑ Fraction of inspired oxygen	↑	No effect
↑ Flow	↑ (minimal effect)	↓ (minimal effect)

P_aO_2 = arterial oxygen tension, P_aCO_2 = arterial carbon dioxide tension

The actual mechanism of gaseous exchange in high frequency ventilation is not entirely understood, but a vibrating diaphragm with a constant flow of gas delivers the breaths providing active inspiration and expiration. Breathing rates/frequency are expressed in hertz (Hz).

$$1 \, Hz = 1 \, breath/s = 60 \, breaths/min.$$

Frequencies of 10–15 Hz are often used = 600–900 breaths per minute.

Oscillatory amplitude (difference between peak and trough pressure) directly determines tidal volumes delivered.

Ventilator setting and recording for high frequency oscillation ventilation

Parameters that need to be set and recorded hourly or according to local hospital policy include: F_iO_2, MAP, oscillatory amplitude (ΔP) breath frequency (Hz), inspired time (IT) and flow. It is very difficult to generalise but, as a guide, figures that might be used as a starting point for a child requiring oscillation ventilation when conventional ventilation has failed are given in the box below.

An X-ray should be taken to assess the recruitment of lung volume once the child is on the oscillator. Usually the F_iO_2 is weaned first until it reaches 0.4 and only then will the pressures be reduced.

If using the SLE 2000 ventilator in HFO mode, the amplitude peak inspiratory pressure, mean airways pressure, positive end expiratory pressure, inspired time, rate, patient's own rate, humidifier temperature and the fraction of inspired oxygen should be recorded hourly or according to local

---

Box 2.3 Setting up for use with Sensor Medics high-frequency oscillator

MAP	Up to 8 cm H_2O above MAP on conventional ventilator
ΔP	Depends on the characteristics of the chest wall and MAP required, but ΔP or oscillatory amplitude should be sufficient to cause subjective chest oscillation
Hz	8–10 (this could be as low as 6 for an older child and up to 12 for an infant)
Inspired time	33%
Flow (L/min)	20
F_iO_2	1.0 initially

policy. HFO can be superimposed onto a positive pressure ventilator rate, in which case all the usual ventilator parameters will also need to be recorded.

Algorithms for ventilatory management on HFOV are given in Tables 2.5 and 2.6.

NB There will be no distinct inspiratory and expiratory chest movement when using high-frequency ventilation, but rather a chest flutter. It is difficult to identify inspiration, and breath sounds will be high-pitched. Trapping of gas may occur with high frequency ventilation and will lead to decreased compliance and CO_2 retention.

Nitric oxide may be used in the circuit if required. The patient will still require suction and assessment of secretions (Hazinski 1992).

Table 2.5 Management of oxygenation on HFOV considering P_aO_2 and lung compliance (reproduced with permission from Avila et al 1994, adapted from HFO Study Group 1993)

If P_aO_2 is:	Lung inflation	Primary action	Secondary action
Increased	↑	↓ MAP	↓ F_iO_2
Increased	Normal	↓ F_iO_2	–
Increased	↓	↑ MAP	↓ F_iO_2
Normal	↑	↓ MAP	–
Normal	Normal	–	–
Normal	↓	↑ MAP	–
Decreased	↑	↓ MAP	↑ F_iO_2
Decreased	Normal	↑ F_iO_2	–
Decreased	↓	↑ MAP	↑ F_iO_2

Table 2.6 Management of ventilation and action to take to rectify P_aCO_2 (reproduced with permission from Avila et al 1994, adapted from HFO Study Group 1993)

P_aCO_2	Primary action	Secondary action
Increased	↑ oscillation amplitude	↓ frequency
Normal	–	–
Decreased	↓ oscillation amplitude	↑ frequency

METHAEMOGLOBINAEMIA

Methaemoglobin is abnormal haemoglobin in which the iron molecule is oxidised to the ferric state (Fe^{3+}) rather than the normal ferrous state (Fe^{2+}), and this means that the molecule is incapable of binding to oxygen and can lead to cyanosis (Curry 1982, Goldfrank et al 1985). Methaemoglobinaemia may be congenital or acquired. Acquired methaemoglobinaemia is the most common form, where exposure to certain drugs or chemicals increase the rate of oxidation so that it exceeds the rate of reduction by methaemoglobin reductase systems and methaemoglobinaemia may occur.

Methaemoglobinaemia can also occur as a result of nitric oxide therapy, as nitric oxide binds to haemoglobin to produce methaemoglobin. During nitric oxide therapy, blood should be routinely tested to measure levels of methaemoglobin.

Normal methaemoglobin level < 1%. Methaemoglobinaemia should be suspected (Pow 1997) if:

- cyanosis fails to respond to oxygen therapy (Goldfrank et al 1985)
- Po_2 is normal or elevated in the presence of decreased measured oxygen saturation (Goldfrank et al 1985)
- blood is brown in colour and remains dark on aeration (Mansouri 1985).

CARBOXYHAEMOGLOBIN

Carbon monoxide is a toxic, odourless gas produced by car exhausts and fires, among other causes. Carbon monoxide has a greater affinity for haemoglobin than oxygen and when bound to haemoglobin forms carboxyhaemoglobin. This impairs oxygen transport, produces decreased oxygen delivery and tissue hypoxia, and can result in metabolic acidosis if carbon monoxide levels are high. Levels of carboxyhaemoglobin above 60% are often fatal (Hazinski 1992).

NASAL INTUBATION

Step-by-step guide to nasal intubation

- Prepare all equipment prior to starting intubation
- Ensure oxygen and suction are to hand and in working order
- Monitor heart rate and oxygen saturations if possible, as the process of intubation may induce bradycardia and hypoxia

---

Box 2.4   Equipment required for nasal intubation

- Laryngoscope and appropriate blade:
  - Neonate – small, straight blade
  - Young child – small, curved blade
  - Older child – large, curved blade
- Magill's forceps, appropriate size
- Yanker sucker and suction – to gauge appropriate size: size of ET tube used × 2 = French gauge of catheter required
- Rebreathe circuit or Ambu bag – appropriate size
- Oxygen supply
- Introducer stylet: S, M or L
- Endotracheal tube
  - correct size +
  - spare tube of same size +
  - spare tube one size smaller
- Tungstall connector
  - same size as ET tube +
  - spare tungstall in smaller size
- Micromount connector – attaches to tungstall connector
- Nasogastric tube
- Assorted tapes if oral intubation +
  - Duoderm to protect skin
- Drugs prior to intubation according to prescription

Box 2.5   Common doses used for intubation (check local policy)

Ketamine 1–2 mg/kg
Atracurium 0.3–0.6 mg/kg
Morphine 0.1 mg/kg
Etomidate 0.3 mg/kg
Thiopentone 2–7 mg/kg

- If not an emergency situation, pass a nasogastric tube prior to intubation

- Position patient and preoxygenate in 100% oxygen

- Give drugs/anaesthetic agents if required, e.g. ketamine, atracurium etc.

- Doctor will use laryngoscope to visualise vocal cords and use Yanker sucker to clear airway, then will pass oral endotracheal tube initially to judge both size and length

- Resume ventilation

- Cut endotracheal tube for nasal use to correct length and attach tungstall connector if being used. (Blue line on ET tube goes in line with the flat side of the tungstall connector.) The black marking at the end of the ET tube should sit at the level of the vocal cords or, if a cuffed tube is used, the cuff should sit just below the vocal cords

- Cut all tapes as required; e.g. if nasal intubation with tungstall:
  - One thin Granuflex square to protect skin on forehead
  - Two foam squares that sit on top of the Granuflex and sandwich the hoop end of the tungstall
  - Two thin Granuflex strips to protect the cheeks
  - Two thin strips of zinc oxide tape to secure tungstall at nose to cheek
  - A headband of appropriate size for child, double-sided so that it does not stick to the child's head
  - Other appropriate tapes if other methods of securing ET tube are used, e.g. Melbourne strapping or 'trouser leg' tapes to stick to face and tube

- When nasal tube passed, remove oral tube on doctors request, connect to micromount connection or other appropriate connector and resume ventilation

- Observe and auscultate chest for equal, bilateral chest movement and sounds to determine correct placement of ET tube.

- If so, secure tube with tapes.

- Chest X-ray as soon as possible to reconfirm position.

- Preoxygenate prior to suctioning.

Orotracheal intubation is the preferred method in resuscitation as it is quicker than nasal intubation.

Selection of endotracheal tube

Box 2.6   Formula for calculating tube requirements

$$\text{Endotracheal tube size (mm)} = \frac{\text{Age (years)}}{4} + 4$$

$$\text{Oral length (cm)} = \frac{\text{Age (years)}}{2} + 12$$

$$\text{Nasal length (cm)} = \frac{\text{Age (years)}}{2} + 15$$

Table 2.7 Endotracheal tube – sizes and lengths (reproduced with permission from Shann 1996)

Age	Weight (kg)	Internal diameter (mm)	At lips (cm)	At nose (cm)
Newborn	1–3	3.0	6–8.5	7.5–10.5
Newborn	3.5	3.5	9	11
3 months	6	3.5	10	12
1 year	10	4.0	11	14
2 years	12	4.5	12	15
3 years	14	4.5	13	16
4 years	16	5.0	14	17
6 years	20	5.5	15	19
8 years	24	6.0	16	20
10 years	30	6.5	17	21
12 years	38	7.0	18	22
14 years	50	7.5	19	23

Below 8 years of age, an uncuffed tube is used, as the larynx at the level of the cricoid cartilage is the narrowest point and will form a natural seal. After the age of 8 years, the cricoid larynx becomes wider and a cuff may be required to prevent air leakage at this level.

USE OF INHALED NITRIC OXIDE

Nitric oxide (NO) is a powerful pulmonary vasodilator that has specific action and does not cause systemic hypotension. It can be used in patients who have reversible pulmonary hypertension and/or ventilation perfusion mismatch, e.g. neonates with persistent pulmonary hypertension of the neonate (PPHN), children with congenital heart disease and pulmonary hypertension, or children with acute respiratory distress syndrome (ARDS).

Nitric oxide must be prescribed. A common starting dose of nitric oxide would be 5 parts per million and this may be increased as prescribed to a top therapeutic dose of around 20 parts per million; however, regulation of this is sometimes difficult.

In addition to normal observations and blood tests, when using nitric oxide, blood levels of nitrogen dioxide (NO_2) and methaemoglobin should be tested and both, ideally, should be below 1%. (Methaemoglobin levels should be taken 12–24-hourly.)

NO cylinders should be checked regularly to ensure that they do not run out. Infants and children can become very dependent on NO and the rebound effect if the NO supply failed could be fatal.

Analysers must be used to measure NO and NO_2 concentrations.

Scavenger systems can be used, i.e. a charcoal filter can be placed on the exhaust of the ventilator, which gets rid of NO and NO_2 from the circuit.

A circuit should be set up to hand-ventilate the child with NO if s/he is particularly sensitive to it.

Closed-circuit suction should be considered if the child is very sensitive to NO. If normal suction is used, consider giving extra breaths using the manual breath button on the ventilator prior to suction. Record NO concentration hourly on the ITU chart.

REFERENCES

Avila K, Mazza L, Morgan-Trujillo L 1994 High frequency oscillatory ventilation: a nursing approach to bedside care. Neonat Netw 13(5): 23–30

Blumer J L 1990 A practical guide to paediatric intensive care, 3rd edn. C V Mosby, St Louis, MO

Curry S 1982 Methaemoglobinaemia. Ann Emerg Med 11(4): 214–221

Easterbrook P 1994 Basic medical sciences for MRCP Part 1. Churchill Livingstone, Edinburgh: p 137–139

Goldfrank L R, Price D, Kirstein R H 1985 Goldfrank's toxicological emergencies, 3rd edn. Appleton & Lange, Norwalk, CT

Hazinski M F (ed) 1992 Nursing care of the critically ill child, 2nd edn. Mosby Year Book, St Louis, MO

HFO Study Group 1993 Randomised study of high frequency oscillation ventilation in infants with severe respiratory distress syndrome. J Pediat 122(4): 609–619

Hinds C J, Watson D 1996 Intensive care, 2nd edn. W B Saunders, London

Mansouri A 1985 Review: methaemoglobinaemia. Am J Med Sci 289(5): 200–208

Miller M J, Martin R J, Carlo W A et al 1985 Oral breathing in newborn infants. J Pediat 107: 465

Miller M J, Carlo W A, Strohl K P, Fanaroff A A, Martin R J 1986 Effect of maturation on oral breathing in sleeping premature infants. J Pediat 109(3): 515–519

Niederer P F, Leuthold R, Bush E H, Spahn D R, Schmid E R 1994 High frequency ventilation: oscillatory dynamics. Crit Care Med 22(9): S58–S64

Pow J 1997 Methaemoglobinaemia: an unusual blue boy. Paediat Nurs 9(10): 24–25

Shann F 1996 Drug doses, 9th edn. Intensive Care Unit, Royal Children's Hospital, Parkville, Victoria

Siemens Medical Engineering 1993 System SV300, 1st English edn. Life Support Systems, Sweden

Taylor M B, Whitwam J G 1986 The current status of pulse oximetry. Anaesthesia 41: 943–949

Tortora G J, Anagnostakos N P 1984 Principles of anatomy and physiology, 4th edn. Harper, Sydney, NSW

CARDIAC CARE

3

FETAL CIRCULATION

The fetal circulation differs anatomically and physiologically from the postnatal circulation:

- Blood oxygenation takes place in the placenta.

- The fetus is relatively hypoxaemic, with O_2 saturation of 60–70%.

- Tissue hypoxia does not occur because fetal cardiac output is so high – approx. 400–500 mL/kg/min (Hazinski 1992) – and because fetal haemoglobin has a high oxygen-carrying capacity.

- The fetal circulation is designed to deliver the best oxygenated blood to the fetal brain and allow blood to be diverted away from the pulmonary circulation.

- Fetal systemic vascular resistance (SVR) is low – nearly half of all descending aortic blood flow enters the placenta, which provides little resistance to blood flow.

- Fetal pulmonary vascular resistance (PVR) is very high – the lungs are fluid-filled and the resultant alveolar hypoxia contributes to intense pulmonary vasoconstriction. This results in blood flowing away from the lungs towards the low resistance of the placenta (Fig. 3.1).

- Oxygenated blood enters the fetus via the umbilical vein → ductus venosus, bypassing the hepatic circulation which flows into the inferior vena cava (IVC).

- The blood enters the right atrium and flows across the foramen ovale into the left atrium.

- The blood then enters the left ventricle → ascending aorta → perfuses the head and upper extremities.

- The lower part of the fetal body is perfused by a small amount of the well-oxygenated blood flowing from the ascending aorta and a proportionately large amount of poorly oxygenated blood from the patent ductus arteriosus (PDA).

- Venous blood from the head and upper extremities returns via the SVC → right atrium → right ventricle → pulmonary artery.

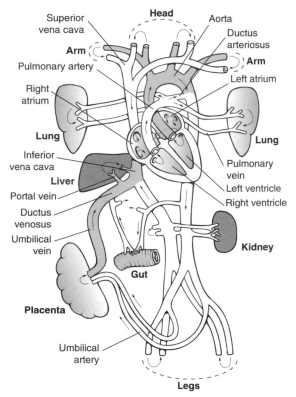

Fig. 3.1 Blood flow through the fetal circulation (reproduced with permission from Williams & Asquith 2000)

- Because of the high PVR this blood flows → PDA → ascending aorta as above. Much of this flow will then return to the placenta via the umbilical arteries.

Changes in the fetal circulation at birth

- When the baby starts breathing, the PVR falls; the increase in O_2 and negative intrathoracic pressure divert blood to the lungs and away from the PDA, causing it to constrict and subsequently close.

- Because of increased pulmonary blood flow, pressure in the left atrium is increased and raised above that of the right atrium, causing the flap valve of the PFO to close. (It can be reopened if necessary by, for example, balloon septostomy.)
- When the umbilical cord is clamped, the ductus venosus constricts and closes.

THE NORMAL HEART

Figure 3.2 illustrates blood flow through the normal heart.

- Venous blood enters the right atrium via the superior vena cava (SVC) – from the head and the upper body – and the IVC – from the lower body.
- Blood flows from the right atrium through a tricuspid valve into the right ventricle.
- The right ventricle pumps the blood through the pulmonary valve into the pulmonary artery and then to the lungs to be oxygenated. The main trunk of the pulmonary artery divides into two – right and left pulmonary arteries – to supply each lung separately.

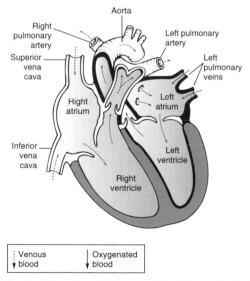

Fig. 3.2 Blood flow through the normal heart (reproduced with permission from Wilson 1987)

- From the lungs the oxygenated blood flows to the left atrium via the pulmonary veins.
- From the left atrium the blood flows into the left ventricle through the mitral valve.
- The left ventricle pumps the oxygenated blood through the aortic valve into the ascending aorta and from there to the systemic circulation.

CLASSIFICATION OF CONGENITAL HEART DISEASE

Children with congenital heart defects have been divided into two categories with a clinical sign, cyanosis, being used as the distinguishing factor dividing the anomalies into cyanotic and acyanotic defects.

The haemodynamic classification identifies different characteristic blood flow patterns. This classification is

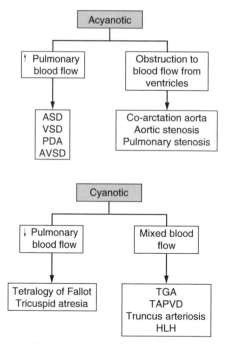

Fig. 3.3 Classification of congenital heart disease (adapted with permission from Whaley & Wong 1991)

frequently used, because of the complexity and variability of the clinical manifestations of some defects (Fig. 3.3).

Acyanotic defects with increased pulmonary blood flow

ASD (atrial septal defect)
A hole in the atrial septum.

Effect: Blood shunts Left → Right.

Management: Closed by cardiac catheter 'umbrella' procedure or surgically – patch repair involving bypass surgery.

Post-op: Possibility of atrial arrhythmias.

VSD (ventricular septal defect)
A hole in the ventricular septum.

Effect: Blood shunts Left → Right; therefore if large, greatly increased flow to lungs. NB If pulmonary stenosis is present, flow may be Right → Left.

Management:

- *Palliative* – pulmonary artery (PA) banding to restrict flow to the lungs.
- *Corrective* – patch repair to VSD and remove PA band, involving bypass surgery. If small, some centres may close VSD via cardiac catheter 'umbrella' procedure.

Post-op: Possibility of residual leak across patch; conduction problems – various degrees of heart block.

PDA (patent ductus arteriosus)
Persistence of this duct beyond the perinatal period – usually closes spontaneously within hours of birth.

Effect: Blood flows from the aorta through the PDA to the pulmonary artery – therefore there is increased flow to the lungs.

 With some complex cardiac defects, it is imperative that the ductus arteriosus is kept patent in order to maintain pulmonary blood flow (e.g. pulmonary atresia) or systemic blood flow (e.g. coarctation of aorta/hypoplastic left heart). Prostaglandin E_2 infusion will be set up in order to maintain a PDA (see Chapter 10).

Management: Closed by cardiac catheter 'umbrella' procedure or surgically ligated – thoracotomy approach. In the preterm infant, indomethacin (prostaglandin synthetase inhibitor) may be used to close the PDA.

Atrioventricular septal defect (endocardial cushion defect)

Openings in both the atrial and ventricular septa.

Effect: Mixing of oxygenated and deoxygenated blood at both levels. May result in atrioventricular valve regurgitation, congestive cardiac failure and left to right shunt with pulmonary hypertension.

Management:

- *Palliative* – pulmonary artery banding to reduce flow to the lungs.
- *Corrective* – bypass surgery to perform patch closures to ASD and VSD and reconstruct clefts of atrioventricular valves if necessary.

Post-op: Possibility of arrhythmias (particularly SVT), degree of cardiac failure due to valve incompetence, pulmonary hypertension.

Acyanotic defects with obstructed blood flow

Coarctation of aorta

Severe narrowing of a segment of the aorta.
This may be:

- *Preductal* – narrowing proximal to ductus arteriosus. PDA allows blood to shunt from the pulmonary artery to descending aorta.

- *Postductal* – narrowing distal to ductus arteriosus. PDA allows blood to shunt from pulmonary artery to aorta. Collateral circulation may supply blood from the subclavian arteries to the descending aorta.

- *Periductal* – narrowing located at level of ductus arteriosus. Bidirectional shunting through the PDA may occur (proximal aorta → PDA; PDA → distal aorta).

Management: Surgical correction (not usually requiring bypass) in infancy if symptomatic – end-to-end anastomosis or subclavian flap repair (subclavian artery ligated so unable to obtain cuff BP in that arm). NB There is a risk of necrotising enterocolitis because of decreased mesenteric blood flow. If coarctation of aorta is suspected, perform four-limb cuff BP in order to make comparisons.

Post-op: Possibility of hypertension: recoarctation may occur. Necrotising enterocolitis/acute renal failure may develop, depending on degree to which blood supply was compromised.

Pulmonary stenosis

Narrowing of the entrance to the pulmonary artery due to either pulmonary valve or pulmonary outflow tract obstruction.

Effect: Reduced blood flow to the lungs. The extreme form is pulmonary atresia, where there is fusion of tissues with no flow to the lungs, when a shunt will be required to provide pulmonary blood flow – e.g. modified Blalock–Taussig (BT) shunt: Gore-Tex connection between the subclavian artery and ipsilateral pulmonary artery.

Management: Stenosed area widened by cardiac catheter technique – inflated end passed through narrowed artery – or surgical correction – patch widening of the right ventricular outflow tract (RVOT). Valvotomy if the valve is the cause.

Cyanotic cardiac defects with decreased pulmonary blood flow

Tetralogy of Fallot

Four elements:

- VSD
- Pulmonary stenosis
- Overriding aorta
- Right ventricular hypertrophy.

Effect: Degree of cyanosis depends on size of VSD and degree of pulmonary stenosis which affect direction of blood shunting through VSD (Fig. 3.4).

Management:

- *Palliative* – if pulmonary stenosis is severe, BT shunt prior to total correction to improve pulmonary blood flow.
- *Total correction* – bypass surgery involving VSD patch closure and patch widening of RVOT.

Post-op: Possibility of arrhythmias and pulmonary hypertension.

Triscuspid atresia

Failure of the tricuspid valve to develop.

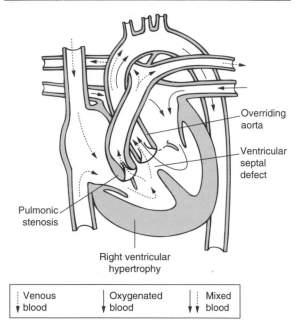

Fig. 3.4 Blood flow through the heart with tetralogy of Fallot (adapted with permission from Whaley & Wong 1991)

Effect: No blood flow from right atrium to right ventricle and therefore to the lungs. The neonate is dependent on other defects (e.g. PDA, ASD, VSD) for survival: TGA may also be present.

Management:

● *Palliative* – maintain PDA with prostaglandin E_2 infusion and BT or Waterston shunt (anastomosis between the ascending aorta and right pulmonary artery) to ensure blood flow to lungs.

● *Correction*: Stage 1, bidirectional Glenn shunt – SVC to right pulmonary artery anastomosis with blood flow to both lungs. Stage 2, Fontan procedure – baffle (tunnel) of IVC flow through right atrium connecting directly to right pulmonary artery where SVC is also directly connected. A fenestration (hole) may be present in the baffle, allowing some escape into the right atrium if the pressure in the baffle becomes high.

Post-op: For Glenn and Fontan procedures, extubate early (positive pressure ventilation impedes venous drainage). Possibility of pleural effusions due to high right-sided venous pressure (Park 1997).

Cyanotic cardiac defects with mixed blood flow

Transposition of the great arteries (TGA)
The aorta arises from the right ventricle and the pulmonary artery from the left ventricle.

Effect: Systemic venous blood returns to the systemic arterial circulation and pulmonary – oxygenated – blood returns to the pulmonary circulation. Survival is impossible unless an additional defect (e.g. PFO, PDA, VSD) is present to allow mixing of oxygenated and deoxygenated blood (Fig. 3.5).

Management. Prostaglandin E_2 infusion to maintain PDA. Balloon atrial septostomy via cardiac catheterisation to improve mixing of blood if septum intact. Surgical correction

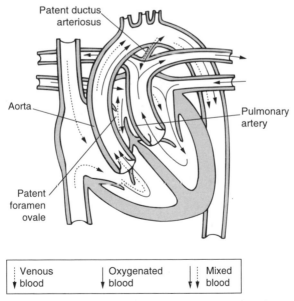

Fig. 3.5 Blood flow through the heart with transposition of the great arteries (adapted with permission from Whaley & Wong 1991)

is usually Jatene (Switch) procedure in neonatal period, where the pulmonary artery and aorta are transposed and the coronary arteries are reimplanted into the aorta in its new location.

Post-op: Possibility of coronary artery obstruction causing myocardial ischaemia/infarction/left ventricular dysfunction.

> Pre-op, if it is necessary to bag the infant, remember that O_2 is a pulmonary vasodilator; therefore use air to avoid unnecessary pulmonary vascular vasodilatation and subsequent pulmonary overcirculation. Consider also the effect of CO_2 – pulmonary vasoconstriction – hyperventilation will lower the CO_2 and again may cause pulmonary overcirculation.

Truncus arteriosus

Failure of normal septation and division of the common trunk into the pulmonary artery and aorta.

Effect: A single vessel arises from both ventricles, straddling a VSD and providing blood flow to pulmonary, systemic and coronary circulation. Four types (Fig. 3.6):

- Type 1 – main pulmonary artery arises from the truncus.

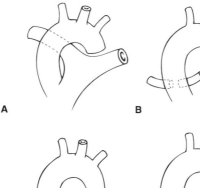

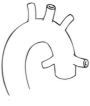

Fig. 3.6 Truncus arteriosus: **(A)** type 1; **(B)** type 2; **(C)** type 3; **(D)** type 4 (reproduced with permission from Park 1997)

- Type 2 – left and right pulmonary arteries arise separately from the back of the truncus.
- Type 3 – left and right pulmonary arteries arise laterally from the truncus.
- Type 4 – left and right pulmonary arteries arise laterally from the descending aorta.

Management:

- *Palliative* – pulmonary artery banding if excessive pulmonary flow, e.g. type 1. Systemic to pulmonary artery shunt to improve pulmonary flow if insufficient, e.g. type 4.
- *Correction* – usually within first few months: pulmonary arteries separated and conduit made from the right ventricle to the pulmonary circulation with closure of the VSD.

Post-op: Possibility of truncal valve regurgitation, ventricular arrhythmias.

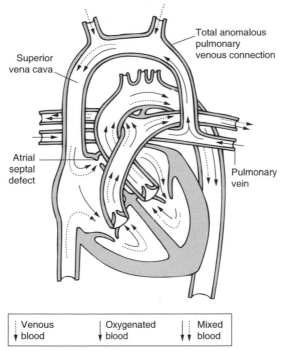

Fig. 3.7   Blood flow through the heart with supracardiac TAPVD (adapted with permission from Whaley & Wong 1991)

Total anomalous pulmonary venous drainage (TAPVD)

Failure of the pulmonary veins to join the left atrium; instead, they are abnormally connected to the systemic venous circulation via the right atrium or veins draining towards it, e.g. SVC.

Four types, classified according to the pulmonary venous point of attachment:

- *Supracardiac* – most common – the common pulmonary vein drains into the SVC via the left SVC (vertical vein) and the left innominate vein (Fig. 3.7)
- *Cardiac* – the common pulmonary vein drains into the coronary sinus or the pulmonary veins enter the right atrium separately through four openings
- *Infracardiac (subdiaphragmatic)* – the common pulmonary vein drains into the portal vein, ductus venosus, hepatic vein or IVC
- *Mixed type* – a combination of the other types.

Effect: An interatrial communication is necessary for survival (PFO or ASD). If there is no obstruction to pulmonary venous return (most supracardiac and cardiac types), pulmonary venous return is large and there is only slight systemic arterial desaturation. If there is obstruction to pulmonary venous return (infracardiac type), pulmonary venous return is small and the infant is profoundly cyanosed.

Management: If obstructed, O_2, ventilation and diuretics to manage pulmonary oedema. ?Balloon septostomy to enlarge ASD. Surgical correction according to site of anomalous drainage – the aim is to channel pulmonary venous return to the left atrium, with closure of the ASD.

Post-op: Possibility of atrial arrhythmias.

Hypoplastic left heart syndrome (HLHS)

A collection of complex defects on the left side of the heart (Fig. 3.8):

- Underdeveloped left ventricle
- Mitral valve stenosis/atresia
- Hypoplastic ascending aorta
- Aortic stenosis/atresia
- Interrupted aortic arch/coarctation.

Effect: Infant is reliant on PDA for systemic blood flow and PFO for mixing of blood at atrial level. Neonates present in hypotensive shock if ductus closure occurs, the inadequate

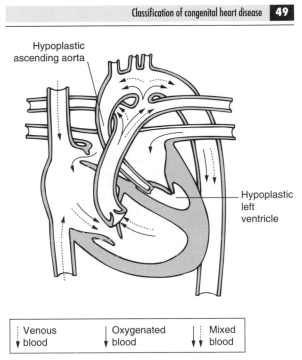

Fig. 3.8 Blood flow through the heart in hypoplastic left heart syndrome (adapted with permission from Whaley & Wong 1991)

systemic blood flow causing a profound metabolic acidosis. Fatal without surgical intervention.

Management. Three options:

- The infant is allowed to die if parents do not wish to proceed with surgery
- Transplantation (not generally considered in the UK)
- Surgery in three stages – the Norwood procedure, which is outlined here.

Pre-op.

- Prostaglandin E_2 infusion to maintain PDA and therefore adequate systemic perfusion
- Aim for SaO_2 75–85% to balance lungs vs systemic blood flow by using room air

- May need to intubate and ventilate – keeping Pco_2 at 5–6 kPa will increase pulmonary vascular resistance and help to keep Sao_2 within desired range
- Correct acidosis
- If infant desaturates, increase F_io_2 but bag in **AIR** if required because of the effect this will have on systemic flow (as discussed above under truncus arteriosus).

Stage One – Norwood Procedure (Fig. 3.9).

- Division of main pulmonary artery and closure of distal stump
- Modified right BT shunt between subclavian artery and right pulmonary artery to provide pulmonary blood flow
- PDA is ligated and atrial septum excised to allow mixing of blood across atria
- Construction of new aortic arch between the main pulmonary artery and ascending aorta and arch.

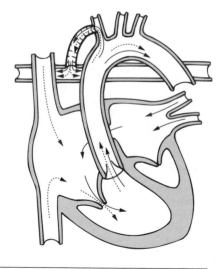

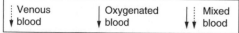

| ⋮ Venous blood | Oxygenated blood | ⋮⋮ Mixed blood |

Fig. 3.9 Norwood procedure

Post-op: Anticoagulation to maintain the BT shunt. Manipulate $P\text{CO}_2$ to balance the pulmonary vs systemic blood flow, e.g. keep $P\text{CO}_2$ at 5–6 kPa and aim for SaO_2 75–85%. (Each centre will have its own protocols.)

Stage Two – Hemi-Fontan/bidirectional Glenn shunt (Fig. 3.10).

- Performed at age of 3–6 months
- SVC → right atrium or pulmonary artery anastomosis with intra-atrial baffle
- Aim is to separate pulmonary/systemic flow.

Post-op: Refer to management of Glenn shunt.

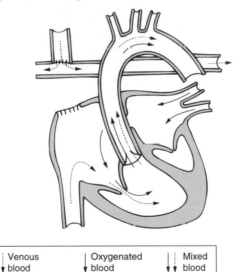

| ⋮ Venous | ⋮ Oxygenated | ⋮ Mixed |
| ↓ blood | ↓ blood | ↓↓ blood |

Fig. 3.10   Hemi-Fontan procedure

Stage Three – Modified Fontan (Fig. 3.11).
Performed at age of 12–18 months.

Post-op: Refer to management of Fontan procedure.

HANDY HINTS FOR POST-OP MANAGEMENT

The goals of post-op cardiac management are to optimise cardiopulmonary support through external monitoring and to

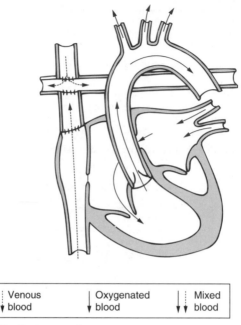

⋮ Venous ▼ blood	⋮ Oxygenated ▼ blood	⋮⋮ Mixed ▼▼ blood

Fig. 3.11 Fontan procedure

prevent secondary injury to the myocardium and other organs while providing effective analgesia/anxiolysis (Papo et al 1997).

Every centre that performs cardiac surgery will have its own guidelines for post-op care – the following are intended as general reminders:

1. Ascertain pre-op anatomy and type of surgery performed. If cardiopulmonary bypass was used, find out the duration of the bypass and cross-clamp time and whether there were any problems related to coming off bypass. Glean any other relevant information from surgical/anaesthetic staff – is there anything else they are concerned about that you need to be aware of?

2. Assessment to include:

   A – Airway
   - ET tube size and length
   - Security of strapping

- Equal breath sounds on both sides of chest on auscultation

B – Breathing

- Colour
- SaO_2 – is this within an acceptable range given the procedure that has been performed? (Confirm SaO_2 with blood co-oximetry measurement.)
- Is nitric oxide (NO) being used?
- Chest movement, ventilation mode and settings
- Arterial blood gas analysis
- Chest X-ray will enable assessment of position of the ET tube, lung inflation, intravascular lines, drains and pacing wire placement

C – Circulation

- Heart rate and rhythm
- BP/CVP/RAP/LAP/PAP and their wave forms, e.g. does the BP waveform look flat or 'damp'? Is this caused by poor cardiac output or a problem with the line itself?
- Drugs – is the child receiving infusions of inotropes/ vasodilators? If so, check the dosage, rate and route and label lines clearly
- If drains are present, confirm position (chest X-ray), label and mark drainage on return from theatre. Most centres discard this total on fluid charts as drainage in theatre and calculate post-op losses only. 'Milk' cardiac chest drains initially and at 15 min–hourly intervals thereafter depending on drainage and local policy, to prevent blockage. Check drains are connected to thoracic suction at an appropriate pressure
- Are pacing wires in situ? If so, label (atrial/ventricular) and ensure that the metal ends are easily available should the child require pacing and that a pacing box is at the bedspace
- If the child is being paced, ascertain the underlying rate and rhythm and check with the surgeon/ anaesthetist that the current settings on the pacing box are correct. A spare pacing box should be available
- Full set of bloods to include full blood count and clotting screen – may need treating
- Blood losses are usually replaced with whole blood or packed red cells
- Abnormal prothrombin or partial thromboplastin times are corrected with FFP and by keeping platelet count within normal limits
- Low fibrinogen levels and other factor replacement can be corrected with cryoprecipitate

- If bleeding is above 10 mL/kg/h despite blood and replacement for coagulation deficiencies, surgical exploration may be required to assess location of bleeding.

Central nervous system
- Assess and record pupil size and reaction to light
- Administer analgesia as soon as child shows signs of waking from anaesthetic
- Consider giving bolus and then infusion – usually of opiates, e.g. morphine/fentanyl; monitor effect
- Muscle relaxants may be required to achieve synchrony with the ventilator (can also help to reduce the incidence of pulmonary hypertensive crisis).

Metabolic status
- Arterial blood gas analysis, mixed venous saturations and serum lactate to check the child is not hypoxaemic or hypercapnoeic and does not have a metabolic acidosis
- Blood taken for an electrolyte screen will enable any necessary corrections to be made and allow assessment of ionised calcium, blood sugar and magnesium levels.

Fluid management
- Maintenance fluids will be restricted (usually half to two-thirds maintenance), initially with added dextrose to prevent hypoglycaemia – check blood sugar level regularly
- Assess urine output – note and discard urine in catheter bag from theatre (as with chest drains); aim for 0.5–1 mL/kg/h initially
- To assess whether fluid management is effective:
  - Assess peripheral perfusion (pulses, capillary refill time)
  - Assess preload via CVP, LAP or both
  - Adequate urine output
  - Assess urea and electrolytes, Hb and haematocrit, urine specific gravity
  - Assess ongoing fluid losses through drains
  - Fluids are usually given in boluses of 5–10 mL/kg, monitoring preload and urine output
  - Nutritional support in the form of enteral or parenteral feeds is usually started within 48 hours of surgery.

CARDIOPULMONARY BYPASS (CPB)

CPB is a mechanical means of circulating and oxygenating the patient's blood while diverting most of the circulation from the heart and lungs. During CPB the blood volume is circulated continuously between the patient and the bypass machine, where it is filtered, temperature regulated and oxygenated.

The main factors involved in preventing complications of CPB are:

- *Hypothermia* – decreases tissue O_2 requirements, providing some protection against ischaemic injury
- *Haemodilution* – the patient's blood is diluted with a crystalloid solution via the bypass machine to reduce blood viscosity and consequent formation of microthrombi
- *Anticoagulation* – heparinisation of blood to prevent coagulation in the bypass machine
- *Cold cardioplegia* – provides local hypothermia when infused into the aortic root and coronary arteries after aortic cross-clamping to induce cardiac standstill.

The risks of surgery involving CPB include:

- Infection
- Bleeding
- Microemboli, e.g. fat, air
- Platelet aggregation
- Cell haemolysis.

PROBLEMS

Cardiac tamponade

Cardiac tamponade after cardiac surgery is caused by fluid collecting within the pericardial sac, which impedes adequate diastolic relaxation and cardiac filling and impairs myocardial function. It occurs if mediastinal drainage is inadequate (hence the importance of meticulous management of chest drains) or if brisk bleeding related to poor coagulation occurs.

An acute manifestation of cardiac tamponade presents with a tachycardia, high CVP, and LAP and hypotension. Bradycardia is a late sign, which usually leads to cardiac arrest. Open pericardotomy is usually necessary to remove the fluid and therefore the pressure within the pericardium.

Pulmonary hypertensive crisis

Pulmonary hypertensive crisis is characterised by an acute rise in PA pressure followed by a reduction in cardiac output and a fall in arterial O_2 saturation. It occurs more commonly with certain cardiac defects, e.g. TGA, VSD, AVSD, truncus arteriosus. Management includes prophylaxis in those at risk by avoiding factors that lead to increased pulmonary vascular resistance, e.g. acidosis ($P\text{CO}_2$ pH – aim for normal $P\text{CO}_2$ or mild alkalosis), pain (ensure effective analgesia and sedation is administered). NO may be used to improve pulmonary vasodilatation.

In the event of a pulmonary hypertensive crisis, treatment includes rapid hand bagging with 100% O_2 and boluses of IV sedation, e.g. morphine/fentanyl, together with muscle relaxants.

CARDIAC OUTPUT

Cardiac output is the amount of blood ejected by each ventricle (in litres or millilitres) per minute. Normal cardiac output is higher per kilogram of body weight in the child than in the adult.

- 400 mL/kg/min at birth
- 200 mL/kg/min within first weeks of life
- 100 mL/kg/min during adolescence (Hazinski 1992).

$$\text{Cardiac output} = \text{Stroke volume} \times \text{Heart rate}$$
$$\text{Preload} = \text{Afterload} \times \text{Contractility}.$$

In order to obtain the 'normal' cardiac output for children of different ages and sizes, the cardiac index is calculated.

$$\text{Cardiac index} = \frac{\text{Cardiac output}}{\text{Body surface area m}^2}$$

Normal range $= 3.5\text{–}5.5\,\text{L/min/m}^2$ body surface area (Shemie 1997).

Cardiac output is a prime determinant of haemodynamic function, and in the critically ill child should be evaluated as either adequate or inadequate to meet the child's metabolic demands.

Preload is the amount of myocardial fibre stretch that is present before contraction and is related to the volume of blood in the ventricles prior to contraction, CVP and LAP

(Starling's law). Frank Starling's law observed that normal myocardium generates greater tension during contraction if it is stretched before contraction. However, fibre length is not readily measured and therefore preload or ventricular end-diastolic pressure is monitored as an indirect measurement.

Factors affecting preload: ventricular compliance, tachycardia.

Afterload refers to the resistance to ejection from a ventricle. Ventricular afterload is the sum of all forces opposing ventricular emptying. A decrease in afterload is often associated with an improvement in ventricular function. Because fibre shortening occurs only when the ventricle has generated sufficient tension to equal its afterload, an increase in ventricular afterload reduces contraction time and thus the stroke volume of the ventricle. It is also related to Poiseuille's law, which states that pressure is a product of flow and resistance:

$$\text{Pressure} = \text{Flow} \times \text{Resistance}.$$

From this equation, an increase in resistance will be associated with a decrease in flow (stroke volume) unless pressure increases. Even a normal afterload may be excessive when myocardial function is poor.

Contractility refers to the strength and efficiency of contraction; it is the force generated by the myocardium, independent of preload and afterload. Contractility is reduced by many factors, including hypoxia, acidosis, excessive preload/afterload, hypocalcaemia and nutritional deficiencies.

INVASIVE INTRAVASCULAR PRESSURE MONITORING

Following cardiac surgery various lines will be in situ in order to continuously monitor the child's cardiovascular status.

Intra-arterial pressure

Intra-arterial pressure monitoring is the only way to continuously measure the child's blood pressure. The systolic (higher) figure is the pressure when the ventricles contract and the diastolic (lower) figure is the pressure when the ventricles are relaxing and filling. The normal arterial pulse contour has a sharp upstroke during rapid ejection, followed by slow ejection and subsequent decrease. The dicrotic notch denotes the end of ejection and closure of the aortic valve. Estimates can be made of cardiac output based on the quality of the arterial pulse contour. Low cardiac output may show a narrowing pulse pressure.

Table 3.1 Information derived from pulmonary artery catheterisation (adapted with permission from Shemie 1997)

Variable	Normal range
Haemodynamic	
Stroke index	30–60 mL/m^2
Cardiac index	3.5–5.5 L/min/m^2
O_2 transport	
Arterial O_2 content	17–20 mL/dL
Mixed venous content	12–15 mL/dL
O_2 availability	550–650 mL/min/m^2
O_2 consumption	120–200 mL/min/m^2

Atrial pressure

Atrial pressure is an indirect measurement of ventricular pre-load. It should be remembered that interpretation of the measurements depends on the compliance of the ventricle and normal functioning of the AV valve.

- *Right atrial (RA) pressure*: Directly measured via RA line inserted during surgery; indirectly measured via CVP line.
- *Left atrial (LA) pressure*: Directly measured via LA line inserted at time of surgery; indirectly measured via pulmonary capillary wedge pressure, achieved through inflation of balloon tip of Swan–Ganz catheter.

Pulmonary artery catheterisation (Swan–Ganz)

A balloon-tipped, flow-directed catheter is inserted into the pulmonary artery to allow measurement of cardiac output (equipped with a thermistor) and right atrial, pulmonary arterial and pulmonary capillary wedge pressures, together with mixed venous saturations (Table 3.1). Pulmonary arterial diastolic pressure may accurately reflect left atrial pressure only when the pulmonary vascular resistance is normal.

Thermodilution is the most commonly used form of cardiac output measurement in intensive care. Through a Swan–Ganz catheter, a measured volume of ice water or saline is injected into a chamber on the right side of the heart and the temperature is measured in the most distal site (pulmonary artery). Mixing of blood with the cold injectate occurs during passage of the mixture through two heart valves and one cardiac chamber. The injection is made via the proximal port of the pulmonary artery catheter and the thermal change is monitored with a distal thermistor. Cardiac output curves are generated and a computer is used to determine the difference between injectate and patient temperature (Shemie 1997).

THE NORMAL ELECTROCARDIOGRAM (ECG)

An ECG measures the electrical activity of the heart and records it on graph paper. This allows the sequence and magnitude of the electrical impulses generated by the heart to be analysed and evaluated (Fig. 3.12).

Information supplied by the ECG includes:

- Heart rate and rhythm
- Abnormalities of conduction
- Muscular damage (ischaemia)
- Hypertrophy
- Effects of electrolyte imbalance
- Influence of various drugs
- Pericardial disease.

The contraction of any muscle is associated with electrical changes called depolarisation, and these changes can be detected by electrodes attached to the surface of the body. Although the heart has four chambers, from the

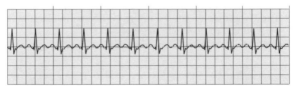

Rate: 120 bpm

A

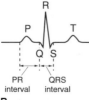

B

Fig. 3.12 **(A)** Normal ECG trace (sinus rhythm). **(B)** Labelled portion of sinus rhythm

electrical point of view it can be thought of as having only two, as the atria contract together and then the ventricles contract together.

The electrical discharge for each cycle starts in the sinoatrial (SA) node in the right atrium. Depolarisation then spreads through the atrial muscle fibres. There is a delay while depolarisation spreads through the atrioventricular (AV) node (also in the right atrium). The conduction is then very rapid down specialised conduction tissue – first a single pathway, the 'bundle of His', then this divides in the septum between the ventricles into right and left bundle branches. The left bundle branch divides itself into two. Conduction spreads rapidly through the mass of the ventricular muscle through specialised tissue called 'Purkinje fibres'. Repolarisation then takes place – the return of the ventricular mass to the electrical state (Hampton 1992).

- **The P wave** represents the contraction and depolarisation of the atria. Their muscle mass is relatively small and the electrical charge accompanying their contraction is therefore also small.
- **The PR interval** represents the time taken for the impulse to spread from the SA node, through the atrial muscle and the AV node, down the bundle of His and into the ventricular muscle.
- **The QRS complex** represents ventricular depolarisation. As the ventricles are large, there is a large deflection of the ECG when they contract.
- **The T wave** represents the return of the ventricular mass to the resting electrical state (repolarisation).

ARRHYTHMIAS

Arrhythmias are deviations from the normal (sinus) rhythm of the heart. Arrhythmias that require immediate treatment in the child are those that significantly decrease cardiac output or systemic perfusion.

There are three main classifications:

- Bradyarrhythmias – too slow for the child's clinical condition
- Tachyarrhythmias – too fast for the child's clinical condition
- Collapse rhythms – ineffective conduction that is unable to sustain cardiac output.

Examples of bradyarrhythmias

Sinus bradycardia (Fig. 3.13)

Characteristics of sinus rhythm are present. Heart rate below 80 beats per minute (bpm) in newborn infants and below 60 bpm in older children may be significant.

Causes: Vagal stimulation, hypoxia, hypotension, raised intracranial pressure, hypothermia, hyperkalaemia, beta-blocking drugs.

Treatment: Treat underlying cause promptly. Figure 3.15 illustrates the bradycardia algorithm.

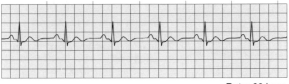

Rate: 60 bpm

Fig. 3.13   Sinus bradycardia

Junctional (nodal) rhythm (Fig. 3.14)

The P wave may be absent or QRS complexes are followed by inverted P waves. If there is persistent failure of the SA node, the AV node may act as the main pacemaker, with a relatively slow rate (40–60 bpm).

Causes: May occur in otherwise normal heart after cardiac surgery, digitalis toxicity, in conditions with increased vagal tone, e.g. raised intracranial pressure.

Significance: Slow heart rate may significantly decrease cardiac output and produce symptoms.

Treatment: No treatment is indicated if the child is asymptomatic. Treatment is directed to digitalis toxicity if this is the cause. Refer to bradycardia algorithm, Figure 3.15.

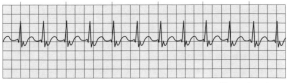

Rate: 120 bpm

Fig. 3.14   Junctional rhythm

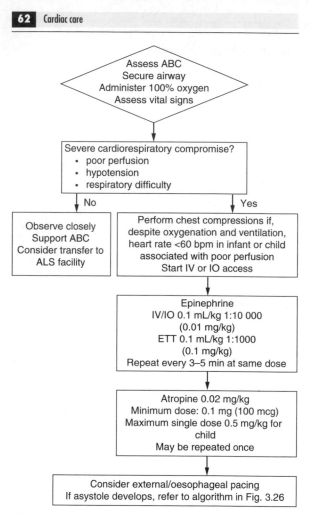

Fig. 3.15 Bradycardia algorithm (adapted from American Heart Association 1997)

N.B. For U.K. guidelines on epinephrine and atropine dosage refer to Table 9.1.

Heart (AV) block

This is a disturbance in conduction between the normal sinus impulse and the eventual ventricular response. It is classified according to the severity of the conduction disturbance.

First degree heart block (Fig. 3.16)
Abnormally prolonged PR interval due to a delay in conduction through the AV node.

Cause: Present in some healthy children, cardiomyopathies, congenital heart defects, e.g. ASD, Ebstein's anomaly, following cardiac surgery, digitalis toxicity.

Significance: Usually no treatment indicated except in digitalis toxicity.

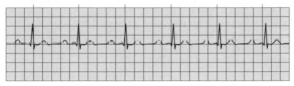

Rate: 60 bpm

Fig. 3.16 First degree heart block

Second degree heart block (Fig. 3.17)
Some but not all P waves are followed by QRS complexes (dropped beats). Several types. A QRS complex follows every second (third or fourth) P wave, resulting in 2:1 (3:1 or 4:1 respectively) heart block.

Causes: Myocarditis, cardiomyopathy, myocardial infarction, congenital heart disease, cardiac surgery, digitalis toxicity, otherwise healthy children.

Significance: The block is usually at the AV nodal level, occasionally at the level of the bundle of His. May progress to complete heart block.

Treatment: Treat underlying cause. Electrophysiological studies may be needed to determine the level of the block. Pacemaker therapy may be required.

2:1
AV block

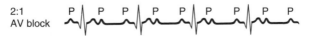

Fig 3.17 2:1 (higher) heart block (reproduced with permission from Park 1997)

R   R   R   R
Complete   P P P P P P P P P P
(third-degree)
AV block

Fig. 3.18 Complete heart block (reproduced with permission from Park 1997)

Third degree or complete heart block (Fig. 3.18)
Atrial and ventricular activities are entirely independent of one another. P waves and P–P intervals are regular at heart rate reasonable for the child's age. QRS complexes are also regular but at a much slower rate than the P rate.

Causes: Maternal lupus erythematosus; congenital type may be isolated or associated with congenital heart disease, e.g. TGA. Acquired type is usually a complication of cardiac surgery. Rarely, severe myocarditis, mumps, diphtheria, tumours in the conduction system, overdose of certain drugs. May follow myocardial infarction. These causes produce either temporary or permanent heart block.

Significance: Congestive heart failure may develop in infancy, particularly if congenital heart defect is present. Children with isolated complete heart block can be asymptomatic in childhood.

Treatment: No treatment is indicated for asymptomatic congenital complete heart block. If symptomatic, refer to bradycardia algorithm in Figure 3.14. Temporary ventricular pacemaker is indicated for children with transient heart block. Permanent artificial ventricular pacemaker is indicated for children with surgically induced heart block and those who are asymptomatic or have congestive heart failure (Park 1997).

Examples of tachyarrhythmias

Sinus tachycardia (Fig. 3.19)
The characteristics of sinus rhythm are present. A rate above 140 bpm in children and above 160 bpm in infants may be significant. The heart rate is usually lower than 200 bpm.

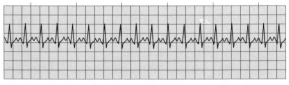

Rate: 170 bpm

Fig. 3.19 Sinus tachycardia

Causes: Pain, anxiety, fever, hypovolaemia, circulatory shock, anaemia, congestive heart failure, myocardial disease.

Significance: Increased cardiac work is well tolerated by the healthy myocardium.

Treatment: Treat the underlying cause. Refer to Figure 3.22.

Supraventricular tachycardia (SVT; Fig. 3.20)
The heart rate is extremely rapid and regular (around 240 bpm). The P wave is usually visible but has an abnormal P axis and either precedes or follows the QRS complex.

Causes: No demonstrable heart disease present in many children. Some congenital heart defects, e.g. Ebstein's anomaly, TGA, are more prone to this arrhythmia.

Significance: It may decrease cardiac output and result in congestive cardiac failure – if this develops, the infant's condition can deteriorate rapidly.

Treatment: Prompt management is required. Vagal stimulatory measures, e.g. massaging the carotid sinus, ET tube suctioning if intubated, may be effective in older children. Placing an icebag on the face on infants for up to 10 seconds has proved effective. Refer to Figure 3.22.

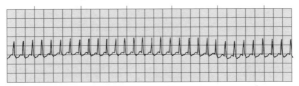

Rate: about 300 bpm

Fig. 3.20 Supraventricular tachycardia (reproduced with permission from American Heart Association 1997)

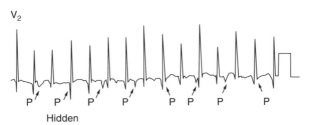

Fig. 3.21 Junctional ectopic tachycardia (reproduced with permission from Legras 1997)

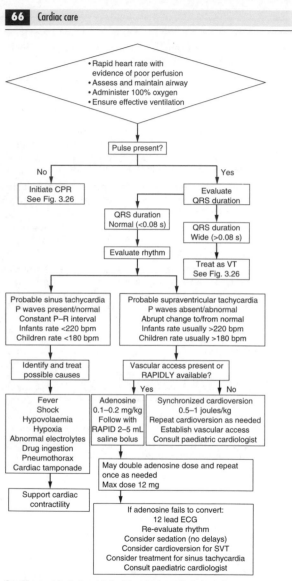

See Chapter 1 for further details of drug treatment for tachycardia

Fig. 3.22 Algorithm for tachycardia with poor perfusion (adapted from American Heart Association 1997)

Junctional ectopic tachycardia (JET; Fig. 3.21, p. 65)

Narrow QRS complex tachycardia with a rate of more than 120 bpm in the presence of AV dissociation; in this case, the ventricular rate is faster than the atrial rate.

Causes: Most frequent in patients with pre-op and residual right ventricular hypertension. Extensive surgery near the AV node with structural or hypoxic damage is an important factor, as are post-op pyrexia and high levels of circulating catecholamines.

Significance: Considered one of the most refractory and lethal of the post-op arrhythmias – does not respond to cardioversion, difficult to treat medically, results in the loss of AV synchrony in patients immediately after complex cardiac surgery.

Treatment:

- Treat hypovolaemia and fever
- Correct hypokalaemia to 4–5 mmol/L within 1–2 h
- Patient should be sedated, paralysed and cooled to 35°C core prior to the use of drugs
- Inotropes should be reduced as much as possible
- Once tachycardia reduces to less than 160 bpm, atrial pacing at approximately 10 bpm faster than JET may provide AV synchrony and suppress this arrhythmia
- Antiarrhythmic drugs, e.g. amiodarone, may be indicated if no response is achieved by the above management
- If all other treatment fails, extracorporeal membrane oxygenation (ECMO) may be useful because JET tends to resolve over time (Legras 1997).

Atrial fibrillation (Fig. 3.23)

Atrial fibrillation is characterised by an extremely fast atrial rate (flutter wave at 350–600 bpm) and an irregular ventricular response with normal QRS complexes.

Causes: Structural heart disease with dilated atria, myocarditis, previous surgery involving atria, digitalis toxicity.

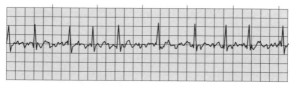

Rate: 100 bpm

Fig. 3.23 Atrial fibrillation

Significance: Rapid ventricular rate and the loss of co-ordinated contraction of the atria and the ventricles decrease cardiac output. Atrial thrombus formation may occur.

Treatment: Digoxin is given to slow the ventricular rate and propranolol may be added if necessary. Cardioversion may be indicated, but recurrence is common. Patients should preferably be anticoagulated for 3–4 weeks before and after cardioversion to prevent embolisation of atrial thrombus.

Wolff–Parkinson–White (WPW) Syndrome (Fig. 3.24)
WPW syndrome is characterised by a short PR interval, and the QRS complex shows an early slurred upstroke called a delta wave.

Significance: Results from an anomalous conduction pathway between the atrium and the ventricle, bypassing the normal delay of conduction in the AV node. Children with WPW syndrome are prone to sustained attacks of SVT (Park 1997).

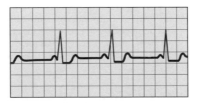

Fig. 3.24   Wolff–Parkinson–White syndrome

Examples of collapse rhythms

It is assumed that basic life support measures to assess and maintain:

- Airway
- Breathing and
- Circulation

have been initiated. Refer to Chapter 1 for further information about management.

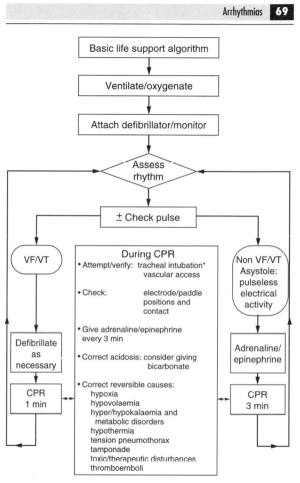

*See Chapter 2 for step-by-step guide to intubation

Fig. 3.25 Paediatric advanced life support algorithm (reproduced with permission from Resuscitation Council UK 1998)

Ventricular fibrillation (VF; Fig. 3.26)

VF is characterised by bizarre complexes at varying sizes and configuration. The rate is rapid and irregular.

Causes: Post-op state, severe hypoxia, hyperkalaemia, digitalis, myocardial infarction, some drugs (e.g. anaesthetics).

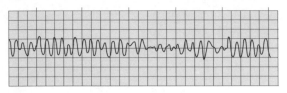

Fig. 3.26 Ventricular fibrillation

Significance: Can be fatal, since it results in ineffective circulation.

Treatment: Refer to Figure 3.25.

Ventricular tachycardia (VT; Fig. 3.27)

VT is characterised by rapid, wide QRS complexes (rate of 120–200 bpm) with an absence of P waves. The QRS complexes are slightly irregular and vary slightly in shape.

Causes: Cardiomyopathy, cardiac tumours, pre- or post-op, congenital heart disease, digitalis toxicity, certain drugs including antibiotics, antihistamines, insecticides and some anaesthetic agents.

Significance: Usually signifies a serious myocardial pathology or dysfunction. Cardiac output may decrease notably and deteriorate to VF.

Treatment: Check whether pulse is present. If not, refer to algorithm in Figure 3.25. If pulse is present, synchronised cardioversion is required at 0.5 J/kg.

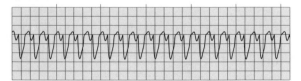

Rate: 180 bpm

Fig. 3.27 Ventricular tachycardia

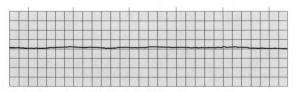

Fig. 3.28 Asystole (reproduced with permission from Riemenschneider 1987)

Asystole (Fig. 3.28)

Asystole is characterised by a straight line on the ECG monitor, with P waves occasionally observed.

Causes: Respiratory arrest, myocardial infarction.

Significance: Diagnosed by the absence of a palpable central pulse accompanied by apnoea, together with absent cardiac electrical activity.

Treatment: Refer to algorithm in Figure 3.25.

Pulseless electrical activity (PEA)

This was previously known as electromechanical dissociation (EMD). PEA is characterised by organised electrical activity on the ECG monitor but there is an absence of palpable pulses and inadequate cardiac output.

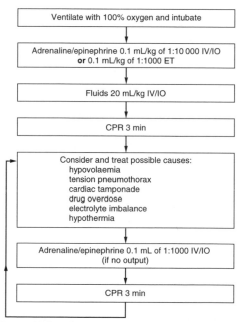

Fig. 3.29 Guidelines for treatment of PEA (reproduced with permission from Guy's, St Thomas' and Lewisham Hospitals 1999)

Causes: Severe hypovolaemia, severe acidosis, hypoxaemia, tension pneumothorax, cardiac tamponade, hypothermia, hyperkalaemia, drug overdose.

Significance: The underlying cause of PEA must be sought, but PEA should be treated and managed like asystole until the specific cause has been identified and treated.

Treatment: See Figure 3.29.

REFERENCES

American Heart Association 1997 Pediatric advanced life support, 3rd edn. American Heart Association, Dallas, TX

Guy's, St Thomas' and Lewisham Hospitals 1999 Paediatric formulary, 5th edn. Guy's, St Thomas' and Lewisham Hospitals, London

Hampton J R 1992 The ECG made easy, 4th edn. Churchill Livingstone, Edinburgh

Hazinski M F (ed) 1992 Nursing care of the critically ill child, 2nd edn. C V Mosby, St Louis, MO

Legras M D 1997 Arrythmias in the pediatric intensive care unit. In: Singh N L (ed) Manual of pediatric critical care. W B Saunders, Philadelphia, PA

Papo M C, Hernan L J, Fuhrman B P 1997 Postoperative cardiac care for congenital heart disease. In: Singh N L (ed) Manual of pediatric critical care. W B Saunders, Philadelphia, PA

Park M K 1997 The pediatric cardiology handbook, 2nd edn. C V Mosby, St Louis, MO

Resuscitation Council UK 1998 The 1998 resuscitation guidelines for use in the United Kingdom. Edinburgh Resuscitation Council, London

Riemenschneider T 1987 The cardiovascular system. In: Behrman R, Vaughn V, Nelson W (eds) Nelson textbook of pediatrics. WB Saunders, Philadelphia, PA

Shemie S D 1997 Cardiovascular monitoring. In: Singh N L (ed) Manual of pediatric critical care. W B Saunders, Philadelphia, PA

Whaley L F, Wong D L 1991 Nursing care of infants and children, 4th edn. C V Mosby, St Louis, MO

Williams C, Asquith J (eds) 2000 Paediatric intensive care nursing. Churchill Livingstone, Edinburgh

Wilson K J W 1987 Ross and Wilson anatomy and physiology in health and illness, 6th edn. Churchill Livingstone

RENAL DYSFUNCTION

Renal failure is the inability of the kidneys to excrete waste products, concentrate urine, regulate electrolyte concentration and maintain pH.

Acute renal failure is the sudden loss or deterioration of kidney function with a progressive rise of serum creatinine and urea. Other characteristics include disturbance in fluid balance, acid–base balance and hyperkalaemia.

> **Box 4.1   Normal values (Guy's Hospital 1999)**
>
> Urea   2.5–7.5 mmol/L
> Creatinine   40–90 µmol/L
> Potassium   3.5–5 mmol/L
> Sodium   135–145 mmol/L

The causes of acute renal failure (ARF) are commonly classified according to the location of the primary disorder:

1. Prerenal – disordered perfusion of a kidney that is structurally normal. Situations causing reduced blood flow to the kidney include:
   - Poor myocardial function
   - Cardiac surgery
   - Reduced blood volume, e.g. trauma
   - Moderate to severe dehydration
   - Septic shock, e.g. meningococcaemia.

   Correcting the underperfusion may correct the renal failure.
2. Intrinsic – damage to kidney function: glomerulus/tubules/renal vasculature. Causes include:
   - Uncorrected prerenal ARF, e.g. persistent shock with meningococcaemia
   - Drug toxicity, e.g. gentamicin
   - Primary renal disease, e.g. haemolytic uraemic syndrome.

   Non-reversible – fluid resuscitation will not improve urine output.
3. Post-renal – disordered urinary drainage: refers to any obstructive lesion beyond the renal tubule. Causes include:
   - Involvement of posturethral valves

- Congenital abnormality
- Related to blood clots, calculi, tumours
- Trauma.

Treatment requires accurate assessment of the cause; if this can be corrected swiftly, intrinsic renal failure may be avoided.

Methods of treating acute renal failure in the critically ill child are:

- Peritoneal dialysis (PD)
- Continuous veno-venous haemofiltration (CVVH)
- Continuous veno-venous haemodiafiltration (CVVHD)
- Haemodialysis.

PROCESSES INVOLVED IN FLUID AND SOLUTE REMOVAL

Solute removal by *diffusion* – the movement of solutes down their concentration gradients, from regions of higher to lower concentration until uniformity is reached.

Movement of water by *ultrafiltration* – the movement of fluid (water) down a pressure gradient, i.e. from a region of high pressure on one side of the membrane to a region of low pressure on the other.

Removal of solutes by *convection* – the movement of solutes with a water flow (solvent drag), e.g. the movement of membrane-permeable solutes with ultrafiltered water. Although the convection associated with ultrafiltration results in some solute transfer, this is primarily by passive diffusion.

Movement of water by *osmosis* – the movement of water through a membrane from an area of high to low water concentration. During osmosis water molecules move across the membrane to the side containing a higher concentration of osmotically active particles.

PERITONEAL DIALYSIS (PD)

PD has generally been the preferred method of managing the critically ill child in acute renal failure but may be contraindicated by an acute surgical abdomen or access difficulties, diaphragmatic splinting causing problems with mechanical ventilation, and catheter malfunction.

PD involves the introduction of dialysis fluid into the peritoneal cavity through a catheter placed in the lower part of the abdomen. The peritoneum serves as the dialysis membrane. This is intracorporeal blood purification as no blood ever leaves the body of the patient.

An osmotic pressure gradient is applied by the addition to the dialysis fluid of an osmotic agent, glucose, which draws water from the blood. The concentration of glucose is chosen according to the fluid removal required.

Solutes are transported across the membrane by diffusion, the concentration gradient being between the blood and the PD fluid. Waste products present in the blood perfusing the peritoneum will diffuse from the blood vessels into the dialysis fluid.

When the dialysis fluid is drained from the abdominal cavity, it contains waste products and excess fluid extracted from the blood.

Fluid and solute removal in PD is controlled by:

- glucose concentration
- dwell time
- volume
- peritoneal membrane characteristics.

Some solutes are transported from the PD fluid to the blood during dialysis – hence the PD fluid needs to contain sufficient amounts of a buffer source particularly important during bicarbonate PD.

Bags of fluid for bicarbonate PD in the acidotic patient are usually made up in pharmacy and ordered as required. An example of bicarbonate PD composition (Guy's Hospital 1999) is as follows:

NaCl 0.9%:	650 mL
Dextrose 5%:	300 mL
Dextrose 50%:	10 mL
NaHCO$_3$ 8.4%:	40 mL

This gives:

Na:	140 mmol/L
Dextrose:	2%
Bicarbonate:	40 mmol/L.

The following details need to be prescribed:

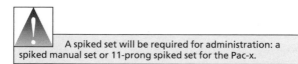

A spiked set will be required for administration: a spiked manual set or 11-prong spiked set for the Pac-x.

1. **Exchange volume** –20–30 mL/kg is generally effective. It will take a longer time for the concentration gradient to decline in a large volume of fluid. In the critically ill child, it may be necessary to use the smaller volume because of

cardiovascular instability. PD can also be of value when used for cooling purposes in the critically ill child with a pyrexia that is unresponsive to other antipyretic therapy. In this instance exchange volumes of 10–20 mL/kg are generally used, with dialysate that can be either cooled or at room temperature.

2. **Fill time, dwell time and drain time** – fluid removal rate is highest at the beginning of each exchange cycle, when the glucose concentration between the blood and the fresh dialysate solution is at its greatest. After a peak is reached, the removed volume falls as fluid is transported in the reverse direction, i.e. from the dialysis fluid back to the blood. If the dialysis solution is kept in the abdominal cavity long enough, the patient will gain rather than lose fluid.

3. **Composition of the dialysate** – bicarbonate dialysate, or 1.36%, 2.27% or 3.86% glucose. The higher the concentration of glucose, the larger the osmotic pressure, resulting in a larger fluid removal. It is possible to use a combination of these different solutions, either by giving 50% of each for every cycle (if manual PD, use burette), or by alternating the different strengths so each is given only on alternate cycles.

Aim to use the minimum concentration of glucose dialysate when possible – prolonged use of the 3.86% solution can result in sclerosis of the peritoneum, making further PD impossible.

4. **Heparin** (500 IU/L) is usually added to the dialysate to prevent fibrin formation and clotting in the catheter. Potassium may also be added, in order to maintain a normal serum potassium level.

Most PD performed in PICU is continuous, and is maintained until the child is able to pass urine and the kidneys are functioning adequately.

Problems

Technical problems with PD are mostly related to catheter malfunction:

- If fill time takes longer than 10 min – it usually indicates catheter obstruction

- If less than 80% of the previous fill volume returns
  during the full drainage period, then drainage is
  inadequate.

Causes

- External kinks
- Fibrin or blood clot plugging
- Poor position or migration of catheter
- Obstruction by omentum
- Leaks around catheter site.

Action

- Reposition patient
- Alert medical colleagues, as catheter may benefit
  from careful flushing with sterile saline; abdominal
  X-ray will confirm position of catheter in
  abdomen
- Fibrin clotting may require urokinase infusion into
  catheter
- Leaks around catheter site will increase the risk of
  infection in addition to impairing the dialysis process;
  therefore medical staff may have to introduce new
  catheter.

In many centres, the Pac-x machine, made by Baxter,
is used for PD – with this machine, however, the minimum
delivery volume is 50 mL, so it may be necessary to use
manual PD for babies whose requirements are less than
this.

In the event of poor flow of fluid to the patient in this case,
it is worth checking the warming coil – some are made of very
thin plastic, which kinks easily and obstructs the flow. These
can usually be replaced without having to renew the entire
circuit.

Full instructions on how to set up and troubleshoot the Pac-
x machine are usually attached to it.

When the machine says the cycle result was positive,
this indicates that the *machine's* balance is positive, therefore
the patient is *negative*.

CONTINUOUS VENO-VENOUS HAEMOFILTRATION (CVVH)

Haemofiltration = ultrafiltration + convection + fluid replacement.

CVVH is the removal of fluid via a semipermeable membrane (haemofilter) using a circuit with a pump. The blood is obtained and returned to the venous circulation; this is an uninterrupted process.

Indications for use of CVVH

- When PD is contraindicated or has failed
- Hypervolaemia that does not require haemodialysis because of improving renal function (urea, creatinine and other electrolytes assessed)
- To ensure that adequate nutrition can be given in suitable volumes, to help decrease or prevent catabolism, and the equivalent volume can be removed.

CONTINUOUS VENO-VENOUS HAEMODIAFILTRATION (CVVHD)

Haemodiafiltration = ultrafiltration + convection + fluid replacement + diffusion.

CVVHD is the removal of excess fluid and biochemical waste products via a semipermeable membrane (haemofilter). Dialysis is performed by infusing dialysate fluid using a countercurrent flow through the haemofilter. The circuit has a pump. The blood is obtained and returned to the venous circulation; this is an uninterrupted process.

Indications for the use of CVVHD

- When PD is contraindicated or has failed
- To ensure that parenteral nutrition can be given in suitable volumes, to help decrease or prevent catabolism, ensuring that the equivalent volume can be removed

- When electrolytes are seriously deranged – particularly potassium
- In certain metabolic disorders, e.g. hyperammonaemia
- When child is not cardiovascularly stable enough to tolerate haemodialysis.

HAEMODIALYSIS

Haemodialysis = ultrafiltration + diffusion.

Haemodialysis is the removal of excess fluid and bio-chemical waste products via a semipermeable membrane (haemofilter). Dialysis is performed by infusing dialysate fluid using a countercurrent flow through the haemofilter. The circuit has a pump. The blood is obtained and returned to the venous circulation.

Haemodialysis is an intermittent treatment; it can be used as a 'follow on' treatment for children who, when critically ill, were receiving CVVHD, and whose condition is now stable enough to tolerate larger volumes of fluid and solute removal being undertaken on an intermittent, e.g. once daily, basis. In other cases its use, as opposed to CVVHD, is likely to depend on the haemodynamic stability of the PICU patient.

FLUIDS FOR CVVH/CVVHD

There are several different varieties of fluid for CVVH. Some fluids are the same in composition but have different names because they come from different companies.

Standard haemofiltration fluid (with buffer, without potassium)

Hemasol L0 (Hospal)
Haemafiltrasol 22 (Gambro)
Monisol (Baxter).

Lactate free haemofiltration fluid (no potassium)

Hemasol XG0 (Hospal)
Haemafiltrasol LG10 (Gambro).

Standard haemofiltration fluid with potassium

Haemafiltrasol 21 (1 mmol/L) (Gambro)
Hemasol LG2 (2 mmol/L) (Hospal)
Hemasol LG4 (4 mmol/L) (Hospal)
Monosol K (4 mmol/L) (Baxter).

It is possible to use sodium bicarbonate solution with CVVH with predilution and CVVHD. This will usually be made up in pharmacy and ordered as required.

Otherwise, a buffer in the form of lactate in standard fluid bags, or as a bicarbonate infusion, needs to be given.

PLASMA EXCHANGE

Plasma exchange is a treatment that is used to treat any disease that is plasma-mediated or plasma-borne, and any disease involving the immune system. The aim of the treatment is to remove autoantibodies, pathogenic immune complexes and inflammatory mediators. The treatment rapidly removes these substances, thereby reducing the effects of the disease processes.

Diseases which have been *treated* with plasma exchange include:

- Haemolytic uraemic syndrome (where there is neurological involvement)
- Guillain–Barré syndrome
- Systemic lupus erythematosus
- Renal transplant rejection
- Myasthenia gravis
- Henoch–Schönlein purpura.

A plasma filter is used for the procedure, and this removes the child's circulating plasma (albumin, antibodies and immune complexes, and clotting factors). During the procedure, the child is given albumin 4.5% to replace that removed. Fresh frozen plasma is also given to replace clotting factors lost. Therefore only the circulating antibodies and immune complexes are removed (Lowe 1997).

The PICU nurse's responsibilities include:

- Accurate measurement of fluid input and output
- Monitoring patient's haemodynamic status and altering fluid balance accordingly
- Pre-warming replacement fluid and monitoring the patient's temperature

- Titration of heparin infusion to maintain optimal clotting times
- Regular assessment of blood gases and biochemistry
- Maintenance of asepsis with the catheter site and the blood circuit
- Maintenance of the blood circuit – acting as a 'troubleshooter'
- Source of information and reassurance to the patient and family.

Problems

- Access difficulties
- Filter clotting
- Infections.

Anticoagulation

Obtain guidance from medical staff about optimal clotting times of the circuit and the patient. The aim is to prevent the extracorporeal circuit from clotting without anticoagulating the patient beyond a safe level.

The patient
Once/twice daily, or as condition dictates, blood screens to include full blood count/urea and electrolytes/clotting screen.

The circuit
A machine to measure clotting times at the bedside is recommended for rapid assessment (Woodrow 1993). Aim to keep clotting time between 120 and 150 seconds in order to maintain circuit patency, and adjust the heparin infusion accordingly.

It should be noted that this method is an estimation only, and the following should also be observed:

- Fibrin and clot deposition in venous bubble trap as clots build up in greater areas of stasis
- Rising venous pressure may indicate clot formation in the venous side of vascular access or venous bubble trap
- Darkening blood circuit may indicate clotting
- Continuous decrease in the rate of ultrafiltration

- Observe the haemofilter for clots, dark streaks or
  areas of gravity separation of the blood into plasma and
  cells.

  Brief written observations on the condition of the circuit
  recorded hourly on the appropriate chart can be helpful.

Heparin

Heparin acts by inhibiting the conversion of prothrombin to
thrombin, and neutralises the actions of thrombin; it is
usually administered at 10–30 IU/kg/h.

Record the amount of heparin infused hourly – this ensures
that the heparin pump is infusing correctly and the correct
dose is being given.

You may need to give a bolus of heparin if you give
blood products, as the transfusion will increase the viscosity of
the blood, which can lead to a decrease in the ultrafiltration, or
solute removal and clotting problems may occur in the circuit.

It is advisable to leave heparin infusing until treatment is
discontinued – this ensures that patency of access is maintained after treatment is discontinued.

Epoprostenol/prostacyclin

An infusion of prostacyclin can be used instead of heparin in
certain circumstances:

- In cases where only the minimum dose of heparin is being
  infused and there is a significant systemic coagulation
  disturbance
- If the child has a low platelet count, to prevent or stop
  heparin-induced thrombocytopenia (Nevard & Rigden
  1995).

  Dose range: 1–2 nanograms/kg/min.

  In adults, dose ranges of 2–5 ng/kg/min are widely used
(Woodrow 1993, Kirby & Davenport 1996).

  Prostacyclin is a vasodilator and therefore may cause
hypotension; its action inhibits platelet aggregation and ACT
monitoring is therefore unhelpful. Unlike heparin, boluses of
prostacyclin should NOT be given when blood products are
administered.

Predilution of the CVVH circuit

Most units using CVVH now recommend predilution. This is used to provide a net increase in filtrate output and urea clearance. By moving the equilibrium point towards the venous end of the haemofilter, it also decreases the tendency of clot formation and should increase the life span of the haemofilter.

Generally, predilution rates start at 0.5 mL/kg/min. For example:

0.5 mL/kg/min for a 3 kg infant
0.5 × 3 mL/min
0.5 × 3 × 60 mL/h
= 90 mL per hour.

The following details need to be prescribed:

- Identification of anticoagulation regime
- Reinfusion/dialysate solution
- Volume and rate of fluid that is to be removed (ultrafiltrate).

Maximum extracorporeal blood volume should be less than 10% of circulating blood volume – preferably 8%.
Total blood volume: 80 mL/kg.
For example:

Total circulating blood volume of 10 kg child	=	800 mL
8% of this	=	64 mL
Clearance	=	less than 3 mL/kg/min
Ultrafiltration	=	less than 5% of wt/min (mL)
Blood flow	=	6.4 mL/kg/min
Therefore, with a 10 kg child, blood flow rate	=	64 mL/min.

When priming lines during setting up filter circuit, heparinised saline (5000 IU heparin to 1 litre 0.9% saline) is generally used.

In anaemic children/those where the circuit volume exceeds the child's extracorporeal blood volume, it is advisable to transfuse the volume of packed cells sufficient to correct the anaemia/provide the deficit in extracorporeal blood volume prior to starting haemofiltration.

If the circuit volume exceeds the child's extracorporeal blood volume but the child is not anaemic, then the blood circuit can be primed with 4.5% albumin.

Filter blood flow is determined by the principle of Poiseuille's law, which, simplified, states:

Pressure = Flow × Resistance

$P = F \times R$.

This means that flow is DIRECTLY proportional to pressure and the radius of the tube, and INVERSELY proportional to the length of the tube and the viscosity of the fluid.

On the Gambro AK10, as neonatal lines have a smaller calibre than paediatric lines, the pump speed *set* will read faster than the speed actually *achieved*.

TROUBLESHOOTING CVVH/CVVHD: GENERAL REASONS FOR ALARMS

Alarm: Intermittent arterial pressure alarm.

Cause: Catheter intermittently sucking against vessel wall.

Action: Turn down pump speed, but not below 3/4 of the maximum rate; consider rotating the catheter 180°.
Remember: the arterial sensor measures negative pressure. An increasingly negative arterial pressure reading indicates that it is becoming more difficult to pull blood out from the 'arterial' line. The catheter could be wedged against vessel/occluded/clotted.

Alarm: Arterial pressure alarm followed by venous pressure alarm.

Cause: Restriction of blood flow pre-pump causing arterial pressure alarm and stopping pump, causing venous pressure to drop and alarm.

Action: Correct, e.g. kinked line, poor position of catheter. Press venous pressure button to start blood pump and keep pressing until light goes out. If arterial pressure alarm comes on again, turn off blood pump and rotate catheter 180°. Restart pump.

Alarm: High venous pressure alarm.

Cause: Restriction of blood flow going back to the patient –

• Clotting in venous drip chamber

- Kinked line
- Poor catheter position.

Action: Check for kinks. Consider clots – try to wash back circuit, i.e. run saline through filter and venous bubble trap to aid visibility. Clots in venous line/filter? Need to change them.

Alarm: Air detector alarm and venous pressure alarm.

Cause: Level of blood in drip chamber fallen/frothing of blood in drip chamber.

Action: Turn off blood pump, raise level in drip chamber by sucking air out with syringe; when safe to do so press air detector reset button, turn blood pump back on and press venous pressure button to restart pump. Keep pressing until light goes out.

In some machines the air detector eye is well below the bubble trap. If there is a just a small bubble by the detector eye, try tapping the tubing to clear it.

The suggestions above are for general guidance only and are not intended to replace instructions in the operator's manual of individual machines.

INTRAVENOUS ACCESS (LOWE 1997)

Children admitted to PICU requiring CVVH or CVVHD generally need to have a Vascath inserted, i.e. a temporary, double-lumen central line to be used solely for this purpose, in order to prevent infection and maintain patency.

Site: subclavian vein or internal jugular vein; right side of neck is generally preferred because of the direct line this vein takes to enter the superior vena cava. A chest X-ray is essential to confirm correct placement prior to use. May be left in place for up to 3 weeks.

Femoral veins may be used if necessary – X-ray not essential prior to use. Do not generally last as long as neck lines and, because of position, tend to become infected more easily.

Vascaths will be inserted using strict aseptic technique, are sutured once inserted and a transparent dressing is usually applied.

Heparinisation

Heparin is instilled into the dead space of each lumen to maintain patency. The volumes required are individually documented on each lumen by the manufacturers – the volume of the venous lumen is bigger than the 'arterial' side.

Usually heparin 5000 IU/mL is used; however in neonates/infants 1000 IU/mL may be preferred – check local policy.

Permanent access

Children who receive regular haemodialysis may have a variety of permanent vascular access:

- Haemocaths (Permcaths)
- Arteriovenous fistulae
- Gortex grafts.

It is **vital** to ensure that this heparin is removed before any form of filtration/dialysis begins, and that the lumen are heparinised again correctly when the therapy finishes.

If these children become very sick, are admitted to PICU and require some form of filtration/dialysis, it may be possible to use their permanent vascular access, unless it is believed that they are septic. As the access site itself may be the cause, new temporary access in the form of a Vascath my then be gained.

Haemocaths are semipermanent Silastic catheters used for long-term haemodialysis. They are inserted under general anaesthetic using surgical technique. The catheters are tunnelled subcutaneously and a Dacron cuff helps to anchor them into place. A chest X-ray is essential prior to use. With meticulous care, Haemocaths can last months or even years. The lumen requires heparinisation as described for Vascaths.

Potential complications of Vascath and Haemocath insertion

- Puncture of the carotid or subclavian arteries, resulting in haemorrhage, haematoma or haemothorax
- Pneumothorax
- Brachial plexus injury
- Cardiac arrhythmias – these can occur if the guidewire has been introduced too far.

Complications due to infection

A strict aseptic technique is of the utmost importance when using vascular access. Factors to be considered include the following.

- Vascular access must not be used for blood sampling or IV infusions, except in emergency situations. Frequent handling enhances the risk of contamination and line-related sepsis
- Blood cultures must be taken if the child shows signs of infection. IV antibiotics should be given without delay – even before sensitivities are known
- Indications to remove the line include a purulent exit site, persistent positive blood cultures, hyperpyrexia and septicaemia.

 For children who have difficult vascular access, it is not desirable to replace these lines regularly. Antibiotics have been installed down the catheter lumens to treat line infections.

Arteriovenous fistulae

Arteriovenous fistulae are made by joining an artery and a vein under the skin. Over time, the vein dilates and enlarges, enabling a good blood supply to be obtained for haemodialysis. Two large-bore needles are inserted and secured in place for the duration of the dialysis, after which they are removed and a small dressing is applied.

The fistula is usually ready for use after 6–8 weeks. Infection is rare if a good cleaning technique is used during needle insertion. Many adolescents prefer to insert their own fistula needles, and are therefore trained to do this by nurses.

Position – The site chosen to create a fistula depends on the size and quality of the blood vessels. A venogram is usually performed to determine vessel size, patency and flow, and where possible the fistula is inserted into the patient's non-dominant arm. The fistula can be formed using either the radial or brachial artery and vein.

Care of the newly formed fistula:

- Check the fistula for a 'buzz' around the anastomosis site to determine patency. This can be achieved using a Doppler or stethoscope

- Observe for bleeding, haematomas and any obvious abnormalities
- Ensure the child's hand and fingers are warm, indicating good blood flow – report immediately if poor blood flow is suspected
- Position arm at body level or elevate slightly if the arm or hands become oedematous
- Maintain adequate hydration, particularly in the immediate postoperative period
- Avoid tight clothing/jewellery/wristwatches on the fistula arm
- Never take a blood pressure on the fistula arm
- Never take blood samples from the fistula arm, except when taken through the dialysis needles before dialysis
- Monitor haemoglobin and platelet levels – if the child is receiving erythropoietin, the dose should be monitored to maintain a haemoglobin level of approximately 10 g/dL, especially if the fistula is being used for haemodialysis. A high haemoglobin may cause a fistula to clot. Drugs may be required to reduce this risk, and may include aspirin, dipyridamole and warfarin.

Gore-Tex grafts – These are formed when a piece of synthetic tubing is used to join an artery and a vein. It is inserted in theatre, and the graft is anastomosed on to the artery and vein. There is a constant flow of blood through the graft, which is needled for haemodialysis. It is then used in a similar way to a fistula. The graft should ideally not be needled until 2–4 weeks after insertion. This helps to prevent infection and haematomas, as well as being more comfortable for the child.

Again, strict technique is used when inserting the needles to minimise the risk of infection. If infection is suspected, the graft must not be used, and the child will be given IV antibiotics until the infection has cleared. A Vascath is usually inserted until the graft can be used again. If the graft remains infected, it should be removed.

RENAL DISEASE

Two renal diseases which may require the admission of a child to a PICU are nephrotic syndrome and haemolytic uraemic syndrome.

Nephrotic syndrome

Nephrotic syndrome is a symptom complex characterised by oedema, marked proteinuria, hypercholesterolaemia and hypoalbuminaemia. Although there are many types of the disease, minimal change nephrotic syndrome is the most common in children.

The syndrome may be classified as primary (associated with a primary glomerular disease) or secondary (resulting from a wide variety of disease states or nephrotoxic agents).

- For unknown reasons the glomerular membrane, usually impermeable to large proteins, becomes permeable
- Protein, especially albumin, leaks through the membrane and is lost in the urine
- Plasma proteins decrease as proteinuria increases
- The colloidal osmotic pressure, which holds water in the vascular compartments, is reduced owing to the decreased amount of serum albumin. This allows fluid to flow from the capillaries into the extracellular space, producing oedema. Accumulation of fluid in the interstitial spaces and peritoneal cavity is also increased by an overproduction of aldosterone, which causes retention of sodium. There is increased susceptibility to infection because of decreased gamma-globulin.

Management is aimed at:

- Restoration or maintenance of adequate circulating blood volume and systemic perfusion
- Maintenance of fluid and electrolyte balance
- Minimising glomerular damage and maximising renal function
- Ensuring patient comfort and preventing infection.

Steroid therapy is usually prescribed as this appears to affect the basic disease process in addition to controlling oedema.

> ⚠ Urine specific gravity will be falsely elevated in the presence of proteinuria or with the administration of osmotic diuretics. Urine osmolality is believed to be the best indicator of renal function because it reflects renal concentrating ability and is not affected by the presence of large molecules in the urine (Brunner & Suddarth 1991).

Haemolytic uraemic syndrome (HUS)

HUS is the association of an acute haemolytic anaemia, thrombocytopenia and acute renal failure. This syndrome is one of the most common causes of acute renal failure in children. It often follows a gastrointestinal illness or, in older children, an upper respiratory illness.

Coxsackieviruses and, more commonly, *Escherichia coli* 0157 have been isolated from HUS patients.

- The main site of injury is believed to be the endothelial lining of the small arteries and arterioles, particularly in the kidney
- The intravascular deposition of platelets and fibrin results in partial or complete occlusion of the small arterioles and capillaries in the kidney
- As a result of passing through these vessels, it is believed that erythrocytes are damaged, removed from the circulation by the spleen, and their life span reduced, resulting in a severe, progressive anaemia
- Thrombocytopenia may be present, possibly caused by the aggregation, consumption or destruction of platelets within the kidney
- HUS is associated with damage to the glomerular endothelial cells. As a result, renal blood flow and glomerular filtration rate can be reduced in a degree proportional to the glomerular injury
- Cortical necrosis may be produced by renal ischaemia, and renal tubular damage may be seen. While much of this damage is reversible, recurrences can occur, or progressive renal failure may develop
- Central nervous system involvement may be evident. Irritability, seizures, abnormal posturing, hemiparesis or hypertensive encephalopathy may develop. It is believed that the development of neurological symptoms, particularly coma, is associated with a poor prognosis.

Management is aimed at:

- Achieving and maintaining correct fluid and electrolyte balance
- Blood transfusions as required
- Treatment of anuria or oliguric renal failure may require peritoneal or haemodialysis
- Management of hypertension – hypertension related to hypervolaemia can be managed with haemofiltration or dialysis

- If the child has bloody diarrhoea and/or abdominal distension with decreased gut motility, it may be necessary to be nil by mouth with the provision of parenteral nutrition
- Recognition and treatment of any neurological complications
- Informing and supporting the child and family (adapted from Hazinski 1992).

REFERENCES

Brunner L, Suddarth D S 1991 The Lippincott manual of paediatric nursing, 4th edn. Chapman and Hall, London
Guy's, St Thomas' and Lewisham Hospitals 1999 Paediatric formulary, 5th edn. Guy's, St Thomas' and Lewisham Hospitals, London
Hazinski M F (ed) 1992 Nursing care of the critically ill child, 2nd edn. C V Mosby, St Louis, MO
Kirby S, Davenport A 1996 Haemofiltration/dialysis treatment in patients with acute renal failure. Care Crit Ill 12(2): 54–58
Lockhart K, Lowe R, Harris J 2000 In: Williams C, Asquith J (eds) Paediatric intensive care nursing. Churchill Livingstone, Edinburgh
Lowe R 1997 Introduction to Timbo Ward. Unpublished teaching package, June. Guy's Hospital, London
Nevard C F, Rigden S P 1995 Haemofiltration in paediatric practice. Curr Paed 5: 14–16
Woodrow P 1993 Resource package: haemofiltration. Intensive and Critical Care Nursing 9: 95–107

FURTHER READING

Elixson E M, Clancy G T 1992 Neonatal peritoneal dialysis in acute renal failure. Crit Care Nurs Q 14(4): 56–65
Hutchison A J, Gokal R 1995 Peritoneal dialysis in the ITU: what is its role? Care Crit Ill 11(3): 111–113

LIVER DYSFUNCTION

5

Liver failure is present when one or many of the main liver functions are so impaired that it becomes life threatening. The failure is considered severe when the level of clotting factors produced by the liver is less than 50% and there is encephalopathy (De Jaeger and Lacroix 1997). When liver failure is associated with encephalopathy, the term fulminant is applied (Mowat 1994).

The liver performs many functions, which can be divided into three general categories.

- *Metabolism* – the liver metabolises carbohydrates, fats, proteins, drugs and hormones. It stores the end proteins, uses them to synthesise new proteins or releases them for excretion.

- *Filtration* – Kupffer's cells remove bacteria, endotoxins, viruses, antigens, byproducts of coagulation and other harmful substances from the blood.

- *Storage* – although it usually holds about 600 mL of blood (in an adult), the liver can also contain large amounts during fluid shifts, vascular alterations or other conditions. It also stores vitamins and minerals (Siconolfi 1995).

If the insult is sufficiently severe, the following may be evident:

- Hypoglycaemia
- Hyperammonaemia
- Hyperbilirubinaemia
- Low concentration of clotting factors.

The assessment of a paediatric liver disorder is based on the following:

- Clinical findings
- Biochemistry
- Imaging (Mowat 1994).

A variety of tests measure different aspects of liver failure (Table 5.1) – however one enzyme, alanine transaminase (ALT) is a specific indicator of liver cell necrosis – most ALT elevations are caused by liver damage.

Table 5.1 Liver function tests (adult American values have been replaced by commonly accepted British values. Adapted and used with permission from *Nursing 95 (May) 41, 1995*, © Springhouse Corporation/*www.springnet.com*)

Specific test	Normal range	Levels elevated because of:
Alanine transferase (ALT)	0–55 U/L	Hepatitis, hepatotoxic drugs, cholestasis
Alkaline phosphatase (ALP)	145–320 U/L	Biliary obstruction, primary liver tumour
Gamma glutamyl transferase (GGT)	8–78 U/L	Hepatitis, cirrhosis, cholestasis
Lactate hydrogenase (LDH)	286–580 U/L	Myocardial infarction, haemolytic anaemia
Serum ammonia	40 μmol/L	Renal failure, hepatic encephalopathy, coma
Bilirubin – total	0–22 μmol/L	Hepatitis, jaundice, neonatal jaundice, obstruction of bile flow, infection
Prothrombin time (PT) OR INR	0.8–1.1 s	Vitamin K deficiency, DIC, salicylate intoxication
Activated prothrombin time (APTT)	0.8–1.2 s	Clotting factor deficiencies, DIC
Fibrinogen	2.02–4.24 g/L	

CAUSES OF LIVER FAILURE

These include:

- Inherited/metabolic, e.g. Wilson's disease, galactosaemia
- Autoimmune diseases
- Infective, e.g. malaria, cytomegalovirus (CMV)
- Infiltrative, e.g. leukaemia
- Toxic or drug-related, e.g. paracetamol, cytotoxic drugs
- Ischaemic, e.g. due to sepsis/shock (Mowat 1994).

In the paediatric intensive case unit (PICU), liver failure may more commonly result as part of multiorgan failure in the critically ill child. In some diseases, however, the clinical presentation of liver failure can be unusual:

- Metabolic, e.g. Reye's syndrome
- Infections, e.g. hepatitis

- Toxic, e.g. phenytoin, aspirin
- Haemorrhagic.

Reye's syndrome is a multisystem disease characterised by a severe encephalopathy with a very high ammonia level, together with fatty degeneration and infiltration of the viscera (especially the liver) following recovery from a viral illness. Diagnosis is confirmed by liver biopsy.

THE JAUNDICED BABY

Unconjugated and conjugated hyperbilirubinaemia

Jaundice is caused by abnormally high levels of the pigment bilirubin in the blood (Fig. 5.1). There are two types of bilirubin – unconjugated and conjugated.

Most units have charts where the age/gestation of the infant is plotted, together with the weight and the unconjugated bilirubin level, in order to assess if phototherapy is indicated.

Kernicterus is yellow (bilirubin) staining of the basal ganglia in the brain of neonates with severe jaundice. Acidosis, neuronal dysfunction, alteration in the blood–brain barrier, hypercapnia and seizures are all thought to be contributing factors to the entry of bilirubin to the brain.

Phototherapy

Phototherapy is the use of blue/ultraviolet light on neonates, which causes bilirubin oxidation and destruction. The infant is kept unclothed to maximise the surface area exposed to the light, so appropriate measures are required to prevent heat loss (e.g. covered incubator). Protective patches are placed over the infant's eyes. Insensible water loss is increased during phototherapy and the fluid allowance will be increased accordingly, so accurate recording of fluid balance is important.

Unconjugated bilirubin

- Lipid-soluble
- High levels toxic to the brain – kernicterus

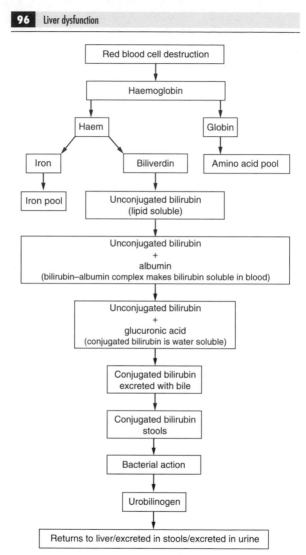

Fig. 5.1 The normal metabolism of bilirubin (Reproduced with permission from McCance & Heuther 1992)

- Responds to phototherapy
- High levels can be caused by:
  - Excessive production of blood cells, i.e. red blood cells breaking up too quickly
  - Immature liver, which cannot conjugate bilirubin quickly enough – cause of jaundice frequently seen in infants
  - Abnormality in the liver preventing the conjugation of bilirubin – rare.

Conjugated bilirubin

- Water-soluble
- Excreted in stool/urine/bile
- High levels can be caused by:
  - Obstruction to flow of bile from liver, e.g. biliary atresia
  - Abnormally small and/or reduced number of bile ducts inside the liver
  - Liver disease causing damage to liver cells, e.g. infection, genetic disease.

A 'split' bilirubin level test measures serum levels of unconjugated and conjugated bilirubin. Jaundice in any baby aged 14 days or over must always be investigated.

ACUTE LIVER FAILURE

Signs and symptoms

- *Hepatic encephalopathy* – staging:
  - Stage I: Normal level of consciousness – periods of lethargy and euphoria
  - Stage II: Disorientation, increased drowsiness and agitation, with mood swings
  - Stage III: Marked confusion, sleeping most of the time
  - Stage IV: Coma
- *Jaundice* – yellow discoloration of the skin, mucous membranes and sclera are caused by excessive bilirubin levels
- *Renal failure* – symptoms are dependent on the type of renal failure: uraemia should be evaluated carefully in the presence of liver failure, as nitrogenous wastes cannot be metabolised appropriately. Increased serum creatinine levels and oliguria are present
- *Coagulopathy* is recognised by an elevated prothrombin time (PT); a PT that is uncorrectable despite intravenous

vitamin K administration reflects significant parenchymal (functioning) disease. Other signs include bruising and bleeding from mucosal surfaces

- *Hepatosplenomegaly* – the liver becomes firm and enlarged, with regeneration, and the spleen becomes enlarged through vascular engorgement. An enlarged spleen and liver, and petechiae, are noted

- *Varices* – with intrahepatic fibrosis there is obstruction of blood flow, with formation of collaterals in the oesophagus and rectum. These veins are thin-walled and prone to the development of varicosities, e.g. oesophageal, GI tract and rectal bleeding (see Sengstaken tube). It is advisable to avoid using rectal temperature probes or administering PR medication to such children

- *Malnutrition* is evident because of inadequate bile salts and the child's inability to absorb fat-soluble vitamins A, D, E and K. Adequate glucose is necessary to maintain normal blood glucose levels

- *Pruritus* is related to bile salt deposition on the epidermis – constant itching can be accompanied by skin breakdown.

Sengstaken tube

A Sengstaken tube is a rubber tube that has two inflatable balloons at the lower end, one of which, when inflated, exerts direct pressure on the oesophagus while the other maintains the position of the tube. At the upper end there are three channels: one for aspiration of the stomach and two for the insertion of air into each balloon. Correctly positioned in the oesophagus, this tube can stop the bleeding of oesophageal varices by direct pressure of the inflated balloon on the submucosa. The gastric and oesophageal balloons are inflated with specified amounts of air/pressure, and are then clamped to prevent dislodgement. Keeping the tube in a fridge prior to use will make it stiffer and therefore easier to introduce. In the event of a child bleeding from oesophageal varices, drugs may be used initially to attempt to reduce the flow of blood. These may include vasopressin, which lowers portal blood flow and temporarily decreases bleeding. Alternatively, endoscopic scleropathy may be performed, which involves the injection of a sclerosing agent either into or around the bleeding varices; the resulting oedema and thrombosis is usually effective in stopping the bleeding. This technique is usually performed by a paediatric surgeon or a paediatric gastroenterologist, and can take place on the unit under IV sedation.

Goals of management

The goals of management of liver failure are as follows:

- Treat primary hepatic injury, e.g. coma, hypoglycaemia and coagulopathy
- Prevent secondary injury, e.g. pulmonary oedema, cerebral oedema, shock, renal dysfunction, infection, pancreatitis and death.

Management may therefore include multisystem support, including the following:

- Ventilation
- Fluid, electrolyte and coagulation correction and monitoring
- Management of cerebral oedema
- Haemodialysis or haemodiafiltration to support renal failure or to reduce ammonia levels in hyperammonaemia (Reye's syndrome/inborn errors of metabolism).

In the event that the liver failure is not part of overall multiorgan failure, extensive laboratory investigations may be necessary to find the cause and to determine whether any specific treatment is indicated. There is currently no rescue therapy in the event of severe liver failure. Transplantation is the only life-saving procedure, and centres that perform this surgery have certain criteria for assessing whether or not it is indicated (De Jaeger & Lacroix 1997).

REFERENCES

De Jaeger A, Lacroix J 1997 Hepatic failure. In: Singh N C (ed) Manual of pediatric critical care. W B Saunders, Philadelphia, PA

McCance K L, Heuther S 1992 In: Hazinski M F Nursing care of the critically ill child, 2nd edn. C V Mosby, St Louis, MO

Mowat A P 1994 Liver disorders in childhood, 3rd edn. Butterworth Heinemann, Oxford

Siconolfi L A 1995 Clarifying the complexity of liver function tests. Nursing May: 39–44

NEUROLOGY ASSESSMENT AND MANAGEMENT

6

In the PICU environment, the nurse is likely to encounter a variety of causes of neurological deficit, requiring careful assessment and management. These include:

- trauma
- infection, e.g. meningitis/encephalitis
- tumours
- cerebral oedema
- neurological conditions, e.g. epilepsy/Guillain–Barré syndrome.

ASSESSMENT

A variety of neurological assessment tools are in use – many are derivatives of the Glasgow Coma Scale (Teasdale & Jennett 1974) or the Adelaide Scale (Simpson & Reilly 1982). The need for the tool to be age-appropriate, i.e. for the neurological immaturity of the child to be taken into consideration, has been recognised, in order to improve the accuracy and validity of the assessment.

An example of an age-appropriate chart is illustrated in Figure 6. 1.

GUIDELINES FOR NEUROLOGICAL ASSESSMENT

- The chart should be used as part of an overall assessment, including vital signs, assessment of fontanelle, if appropriate, and the child's reaction to his/her surroundings and, in particular, to family/caregivers

- Care must be taken to ensure that the pain application, where required, is appropriate and applied for a sufficient length of time to allow a response to be elicited – 30 s is recommended by Lower (1992)

- The effects of drugs that are being administered or have been administered must be acknowledged

- Continuity of interpretation of neurological observations is improved if, during handover between shifts, a joint neurological assessment is executed, e.g. agreement on pupil size

Neurological Observation Chart

Name _____ Hosp. No. _____ Ward _____

	Coded Value	Date Time																								
1. Eye opening																										
• Spontaneous	4																									
• To speech	3																									
• To pain	2																									
• None	1																									
2. Best verbal response																										
• Orientated words	5																									
	4																									
• Vocal sounds	3																									
• Cries	2																									
• None	1																									
3. Best motor response																										
• Obeys commands	5																									
• Localises to pain	4																									
• Flexion to pain	3																									
• Extension to pain	2																									
• None	1																									
TOTAL																										
Normal aggregate																										
0–6 months	9																									
6–12 months	11																									
1–2 years	12																									
2–5 years	13																									
> 5 years	14																									
Pupil size reaction																										
Left																										
Right																										

Pupil Scale (mm)

1 2 3 4 5 6 7 8

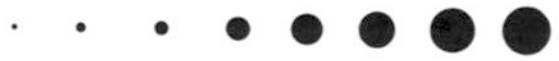

Fig. 6.1 Example of an age-appropriate neurological assessment chart based on the Adelaide Coma Scale (Adapted with permission from Simpson & Reilly 1982)

• A careful explanation of all procedures to be used during a neurological assessment must be given to relatives/visitors in order to minimise distress.

Eye opening

The ability to obey commands is dependent upon the age and compliance of the child.

If the child does not open their eyes spontaneously, assess their response to speech by calling their name, first quietly and then loudly should there be no initial response. If the child is of preschool age and above, ask their to open their eyes. In order to elicit the best response, ask the child's parents, if present, to call their name. If there is no response use a graded sequence of stimulation as recommended by Lower (1992) – shout, shake, pain. The interpretation of 'shake' is intended as a rousing stimulus rather than an actual physical shaking action, prior to the application of a pain stimulus (details below under motor response) to a child who may simply be drowsy.

In order to assess pupils, unless eyes are open, open both carefully and assess size of pupils together – it is easier to see differences when both are viewed simultaneously. The use of a pupil size chart beside the child's face can promote accurate measurement of pupil size. Consider also the lighting in the child's bed space; if it is either very bright or dimmed, this could affect the pupil size when assessed. Interpretation can also differ between assessing individuals.

Each pupil's response to light is recorded appropriately with a + or – sign, and a H for hippus response, which occurs when the pupil constricts, then dilates to light. Note whether the pupils respond briskly or sluggishly. If in doubt, get a colleague to check.

Eyes that are closed by swelling can be indicated by C – if the chart you are using does not specify the above, you could formulate a 'key' for clarification. Note also the position of the pupils, e.g. they may be divergent, or 'sunsetting' in appearance – pupils resemble a setting sun because of downward deviation caused by pressure on cranial nerve III, the oculomotor nerve.

Verbal response

Charts will vary in the age-appropriateness of this category. In the chart illustrated, 'orientated' requires vocalisation of orientation to place, in children 5 years and above. 'Words' is the maximum response for the 12 months to 5 years age group, and 'vocal sounds' includes the most basic babbles and noises for the 6–12 months group. 'Cries' is an appropriate response to stressful situations in the youngest infants – 0–6 months.

Again, involve the parents where possible and take into consideration the child's own stage of development. Has the child reached developmental milestones or are there known delays/deficits?

The inability to produce a verbal response because of an endotracheal or tracheostomy tube is documented as T.

Motor response

If the child obeys commands, e.g. by squeezing your fingers or wriggling his toes when asked, he may also be able to lift his hands and feet off the bed, or push against you with them. This enables you to assess any differences in strength/weakness between the child's left and right sides. Ensure that the *best* motor response is charted, as well as differences; involve parents where possible.

Painful stimuli should be central to avoid confusion with local reflex arcs; pressing the superior orbital ridge, providing pressure to the sternum or giving a trapezius squeeze (to children 5 years and above, because there is insufficient development of this muscle until this age). It is believed that, in the event of no immediate response to a painful stimulus, it should be continued for a total of 30 s to ensure that adequate time is given to elicit the best response. A child aged 6–24 months is deemed capable of localising pain, but from 0–6 months the maximum response is flexion to pain.

In contrast to appropriate flexion there is also abnormal posturing:

- Decorticate posturing – abnormal flexion of limbs to centre of body
- Decerebrate posturing – rigid extension of limbs.

Consider also cough and gag reflexes (endotracheal tube/tracheostomy suctioning and using Yankuer at back of throat, respectively, could be used to test these).

- Posturing – does the child appear to move normally or abnormally?
- Motor responses – any change is likely to be on the opposite side of the problem.
- Pupillary responses – changes usually occur on the same side as the lesion; for example, if a brain tumour is on the left

side, the pupil changes will be on the left and the motor changes will be on the right.

Pupil constriction can be caused by drugs, e.g. fentanyl or morphine. Bilaterally dilated pupils may indicate hypoxia or be due to drugs, e.g. atropine.

A suddenly dilated pupil, or unequal pupils, are warning signs of serious problems.

The hippus response is where the pupils can not sustain the constriction to light and redilate. Bilateral hippus response can occur in meningitis. Unilateral hippus, however, is noteworthy. Hippus response may be normal if pupils are observed under high magnification, *but* it is also observed at the beginning of pressure on cranial nerve III and can be associated with early transtentorial herniation.

The term 'blow a pupil' means that a pupil has become fixed and dilated. This is an ominous sign and requires immediate medical assessment and probably a CT scan.

IDENTIFICATION AND MANAGEMENT OF RAISED INTRACRANIAL PRESSURE

The Munroe–Kellie hypothesis observes that the total intracranial volume cannot expand as the skull is a rigid structure that contains a finite intracranial volume. The intracranial pressure is determined by the total intracranial volume and intracranial compliance (the change in pressure resulting from a change in volume). Skull sutures are not fixed in infancy and can expand to accommodate *gradual* increases in intracranial volume, but not *acute* increases – therefore even in infancy intracranial volume is relatively constant.

Intracranial contents include:

- Brain – occupies approximately 80% of intracranial space
- Blood: cerebral blood volume (CBV) – occupies 7–10% of the total intracranial volume
- Cerebrospinal fluid (CSF) – occupies 7–10% of the total intracranial volume.

Intracranial volume = Brain volume + Blood volume + CSF volume.

If the volume of any of the intracranial contents increases without a commensurate and compensatory decrease in the volume of other substances in the intracranial vault, intracranial pressure will rise.

The relationship between intracranial pressure (ICP) and cerebral perfusion pressure (CPP)

The normal pressure exerted by the intracranial contents is 0–15 mmHg (Germon 1994). Transient increases can be caused by coughing or by moving from a standing to a reclining position, which causes an increase in venous pressure as a result of compensation mechanisms (below). Once the limits of these mechanisms have been reached, significant increases in ICP are seen.

Cerebral perfusion pressure is the difference between the mean systemic blood pressure and the intracranial pressure:

Cerebral perfusion pressure	= Mean systemic arterial pressure	– Intracranial pressure
CPP	= MAP	–ICP

The normal range of CPP in adults is 65–70 mmHg (Singh 1997); 60–70 mmHg is the range commonly used in paediatrics. A minimum CPP of 60 mmHg is thought to be necessary to ensure effective cerebral perfusion – although this is not absolute, as perfusion is determined by blood flow, not blood pressure.

CPP will fall if the MAP falls, if the mean ICP rises or if both occur simultaneously. The CPP can be maintained despite a rise in ICP if the MAP rises with it. This may or may not be associated with effective cerebral perfusion.

Causes of raised ICP

- Trauma, e.g. road traffic accident/blow to head
- Encephalitis
- Cerebral oedema, e.g. infection/trauma/renal problems/sodium imbalance/hypoxia
- Tumours
- CSF alteration
  - increased production
  - decreased absorption
  - pathway obstruction

- Cerebrovascular alterations
  - increased blood pressure
  - vein of Galen (congenital abnormality where artery joins veins in skull).

Compensatory mechanisms
- **Respiratory:**
  - *High* $P\text{CO}_2 \rightarrow$ vasodilation $\rightarrow$ *Raised* ICP
  - *Low* $P\text{CO}_2 \rightarrow$ vasoconstriction $\rightarrow$ *Drop* in ICP
  - *Low* $P\text{O}_2 \rightarrow$ vasodilation $\rightarrow$ *Raised* ICP
  - *Low* pH $\rightarrow$ vasodilation $\rightarrow$ *Raised* ICP
- **CSF:** can be displaced into spinal canal if temperature is high
- **Temperature:** for every 1°C rise in body temperature, cerebral metabolism may rise by up to 19%, leading to a rise in ICP (Fisher 1997)
- **Stimulation:** stress $\rightarrow$ systemic vasoconstriction $\rightarrow$ BP + CBF increased $\rightarrow$ *Raised* ICP.

 Once the limits of compensation have been reached, further increase in intracranial volume will result in a rise in ICP. Progressive small rises in intracranial volume will produce progressively greater rises in ICP.

Clinical signs and symptoms

A child with raised ICP may demonstrate an alteration in the following:

- Level of consciousness – likely to deteriorate
- Pupil reaction – unequal/unreactive/dilated
- Heart rate – decreasing
- Blood pressure – increasing
- Respiratory rate/pattern – slower and irregular
- Motor activity/reflexes/development of abnormal posturing – decorticate (flexion) or decerebrate (extension)
- Response to pain (demonstrating flaccidity).

The child may complain of a headache, or develop nausea and vomiting.

In some instances, Cushing's triad – hypertension/brady-cardia/apnoea – may occur. (This is a late sign.)

X-rays, a computerised tomography (CT) scan or a magnetic resonance imaging (MRI) scan may be taken in order to assist with the assessment of the child's condition.

Management

The goals of managing raised intracranial pressure are as follows:

1. Ensure effective cerebral perfusion through the maintenance of good systemic perfusion and control of intracranial pressure
2. Preserve cerebral function
3. Prevent secondary insults to the brain.

Usually the child will be intubated and ventilated. Central venous and arterial access will be obtained.

Hyperventilation: Opinions vary as to how low the Pco$_2$ range should be kept; some research suggests that sustained hyperventilation (more than 6 h) is counter-productive (Sherman et al, cited by Kerr & Brucia 1993) and many recommend mild hypercapnia – Pco$_2$ of 4–5 kPa (Singh 1997). A Pco$_2$ below 3 kPa may induce cerebral ischaemia.

Fluids: The importance of maintaining a good BP, CVP and CPP is balanced by the need to fluid-restrict and keep child slightly dehydrated, causing high normal ranges in serum osmolality and serum sodium – alleviates cerebral oedema and reduces ICP.

Use of diuretics: Osmotic diuretics, e.g. mannitol (see below), and 3% saline pull fluid from brain tissue into intravascular space. Frusemide may be used to promote diuresis.

- Monitor potassium levels closely – may need replacing.

Position: Conflicting views, but most authors recommend:

- Midline – nose–sternum–umbilicus (Singh 1997)
- Head-up tilt (30°; Feldman et al 1992)
- Support neck laterally – if spinal collar in situ ensure it is not too tight and impeding venous drainage
- Avoid extreme hip flexion – increases intrathoracic pressure and therefore ICP.

Noise reduction: Sudden loud noises can cause a startle reflex – associated rise in ICP.

- Monitors, alarms, telephones – try to silence promptly
- Prevent people talking negatively/airing their concerns about child's condition/accident/prognosis near the bed-space – may cause anxiety and subsequent rise in ICP (Schinner et al 1995).

Drugs:

- Sedation, e.g. morphine/propofol/fentanyl
- Paralysis, e.g. vecuronium
- Antacids if not enterally fed

- Barbiturates, e.g. thiopentone, reduce ICP via a reduction in cerebral metabolic rate and resultant decrease in CBF and blood volume (Singh 1997).

Care:

- Staggering versus clustering – assess child and plan care accordingly.
- Minimal handling
- Minimal physio/suctioning
- Avoid constipation/full bladder
- Avoid rapid changes in position
- Use log rolling to maintain alignment and prevent exacerbation of neck or spinal injury
- Consider bolus of sedation and informing child of all activities prior to carrying them out.

Temperature: Normal or cooled – opinions vary:

- The prevention and aggressive treatment of fever iatrogenic hyperthermia after head injury is emphasised (Singh 1997)

- Cooling to 35°C to reduce metabolic demands and give a degree of neuroprotection in patients with persistently raised ICP is advocated by some authors (Shiozaki et al 1998).

Monitoring:

- Heart rate, BP, CVP
- Temperature, fluid balance.

Neurology: ICP and CPP neuro assessment.

ICP MONITORING

ICP monitoring is a valuable addition to the clinical assessment of the patient. It is extremely helpful in the evaluation of trends in the patient's condition, particularly in response to therapy. ICP measurements should always be interpreted in conjunction with the patient's clinical appearance.

Two methods of monitoring ICP are:

- *Ventricular pressure monitoring* – a catheter is inserted through a burr hole in the skull into the lateral ventricle and is attached to a fluid-filled (or fibreoptic) monitoring system

• *Subarachnoid screw pressure monitoring* – the subarachnoid screw is inserted through a burr hole in the skull and attached to a fluid-filled (or fibreoptic) monitoring system, e.g. Camino bolt.

NB Fibreoptic catheters are zeroed before they are placed, but fluid systems require zeroing on a daily or shift basis, with the transducer being levelled at the outer aspect of the eye.

Hourly charting of intracranial pressure on an appropriate chart should record the following:

1. The average number ICP that hour (the number used to calculate the CPP)
2. The highest peak ICP observed that hour.

This method makes it possible to accurately record trends in the ICP.

Once ICP is stable, there should be a gradual return to normal care, i.e.:

• Increase fluids
• Decrease ventilation
• Stop paralysis
• Decrease sedation
• Continue neurological assessment
• Continue to normalise care until extubation is possible.

Mannitol

Mannitol is an osmotic diuretic, i.e. an agent administered to produce an acute and transient rise in intravascular osmolality, resulting in a shift of free water from the interstitial and cellular spaces to the intravascular space. This free water is then eliminated by the kidneys: urine output should therefore be observed to monitor effect.

Dosage: All ages 0.25–0.5 g/kg initially (Shann 1996). Singh (1997) states that this dose can be repeated 6–hourly if needed, providing plasma osmolality is less than 330 mmol/L. Following mannitol administration, the ICP should fall and the CPP will rise. Mannitol administration in high doses (1–2 g/kg) may increase cerebral intravascular volume transiently and contribute to a rise in ICP (the so-called mannitol rebound effect). This elevation in ICP is thought to develop in dehydrated patients, or in those with a relatively high CPP.

Extraventricular drains (EVDs)

CSF is mainly produced by the choroid plexuses in the lateral, third and fourth ventricles. From these production sites, the CSF fills the ventricular system and follows a pathway incorporating the subarachnoid space.

CSF flows over and around the brain and spinal cord, providing buoyancy and support, and maintaining the constant chemical composition of the extracellular fluid in which the central nervous system metabolic activity occurs. Absorption of CSF into the venous circulation is via the arachnoid villi, which act as one-way valves and are located in the superior sagittal sinus.

CSF is produced at an approximate rate of:

- 20 mL/h in adults
- 5–10 mL/h in toddlers
- 3–5 mL/h in infants (Evans 1987).

CSF is made up of:
- White cells
- Water
- Oxygen
- Carbon dioxide
- Protein
- Glucose
- Sodium
- Potassium
- Chloride.

Indications for CSF drainage

Extraventricular drainage diverts CSF from the ventricles in the brain when the normal physiological mechanisms are unable to do so. It can be used:

- to monitor intraventricular pressure and output of CSF
- to divert CSF that contains bacteria or blood
- in the emergency treatment of a malfunctioning internal shunt and hydrocephalus
- to control ventricular pressure.

Hydrocephalus

This is the result of an increase of CSF within the cranial vault, which causes ventricular dilatation. Types:

- Communicating hydrocephalus – occurs when the arachnoid villi are obstructed and unable to reabsorb the CSF, e.g. in subarachnoid haemorrhage

• Non-communicating hydrocephalus – caused by an obstruction in the flow of CSF within the ventricular system; causes include congenital malformation/tumour (Allen 1993).

Treatment

To treat hydrocephalus, a temporary or permanent ventricular shunt is surgically inserted to divert CSF.

A temporary shunt is a straight, Silastic ventricular catheter, usually placed in the right lateral ventricle through a burr hole made in the parasagittal region of the skull, just anterior to the right coronal suture. The catheter is then attached directly to drainage tubing by an interlocking connector that has an access port. This type of set up is called a simple extraventricular drain.

A permanent shunt is usually in the form of an internal ventriculoperitoneal shunt, where the CSF is drained from the ventricles as above but is then tunnelled under the scalp, neck and chest wall to the abdomen, ending in the peritoneal cavity, where the draining CSF is absorbed (Birdsall & Grief 1990).

EVDs

Several systems are available. Generally, a measuring chamber is positioned to drain CSF at a set pressure through the attached drainage system.

The sets consist of the following:

• Attachment from tubing from scalp to measuring chamber, incorporating a sampling port
• Measuring chamber with bacteriostatic filter at the top
• Tubing incorporating sampling port and three-way tap/stopcock with drainage outlet tube
• Drainage bag with ventilation filter.

Luer lock connections are used throughout for safety purposes.

As always, local policies must be adhered to; however, the following guidelines may be helpful when managing children with EVDS:

• At start of shift check that the drain is levelled correctly as follows:

  – Place the zero point of the scale on the measuring chamber so that it is level with the patient's external auditory meatus – make sure that this is adjusted, and therefore re-zeroed, if the patient's position is changed

– Ensure that the drainage bag is hung below the level of both the measuring cylinder and the patient

• Check CSF for amount, colour, clarity

• Inspect EVD from external site to end of drainage bag, checking all tubing and connections

• Check and document the prescribed reference level of the drainage cylinder, which will adjust the flow of CSF – lowering the reference point of the cylinder increases flow, raising it has the opposite effect. The accuracy of this is therefore very important, and should be recorded hourly as part of the patient observations, together with CSF loss

• The tubing may be clamped for preferably no more than 30 min when the patient is repositioned or transported, during vigorous activity (chest physiotherapy, turning, suctioning) or, for example, when an infant is being held by the parents. Vigorous movement may cause too much CSF to drain, collapsing the ventricles. It is also possible to reduce the amount of CSF drainage prior to vigorous activity by raising the level of the cylinder

• In order to clamp the system, use the stopcock/three-way tap if there is one, or use non-toothed clamps in order to prevent damage to the tubing

• Specimens of CSF are usually taken daily from the sampling port and sent for culture, white cell count, protein and glucose levels

• Hourly measurement of CSF losses should be recorded, commonly these are replaced millilitre for millilitre by normal saline IV

• A protocol of clamping and unclamping the EVD is frequently followed as the child's condition improves, in order to ensure that intrinsic CSF pathways are still functioning, e.g. clamp tubing for 2 h, then open for 5 min and assess CSF loss during that time; repeat four or five times. The patient is carefully observed during this time for any signs of raised ICP. When no more than, for example, 5 mL of CSF drains when the EVD is unclamped, and CT scan confirms ventricular size, the drain may be removed. If the CSF output remains high, or the ventricles remain enlarged, an internal shunt may be required.

COMMON DIAGNOSTIC TESTS

Electroencephalography (EEG)

The EEG is a recording of the electrical activity arising from different areas of the brain.

These areas of activity can be quantified, localised and compared with normal EEGs for the patient's age to assist in the diagnosis of seizure activity or central nervous system injury or dysfunction. An isoelectric (flat) EEG in a non-sedated, non-hypothermic patient is one of the criteria used to confirm brain death.

An EEG is performed using electrodes placed on specific areas of the scalp – the number of these and their positioning depends on the specific machine used.

Computerised tomography (CT) scan

Computerised axial tomography consists of a series of X-rays that are analysed and reconstructed by a computer to produce cross-sectional images. In these circumstances, the X-ray pictures of the skull will produce cross-sectional images of the intracranial contents. The images produced by the scan allow differentiation of intracranial spaces and normal grey/white matter.

The CT scan is a reliable, painless and non-invasive method of visualising a variety of neurological disorders, including space-occupying lesions, haematomas, haemorrhages, hydrocephalus and brain abscesses.

 A higher radiation dose than conventional X-rays is used, but the value of this test is believed to outweigh this risk.

Magnetic resonance imaging (MRI) scan

Magnetic resonance imaging is the application of a strong external magnetic field around the patient, which causes rotation of the cell nuclei in a predictable direction at a predictable speed. The result of the rotation of the nuclei is a resonant image that is extremely well defined and enables the visualisation of soft tissues better than any other non-invasive

 Unlike X-rays or CT scanning, this investigation does not use any radiation. However, it is very important that **no metal whatsoever** is attached to the patient, including endotracheal tube connections and monitoring, because of the enormous magnetic force that is used. It is also very noisy.

device (Hazinski 1992). It is particularly valuable for visualisation of tumours, shunts and tissue or organ thicknesses. The scan also enables detailed visualisation of areas of spinal cord compression following trauma.

Both CT and MRI scans can take up to 30 min to complete, depending on the area which is scanned. As the patient needs to be completely still, it is important that the child be adequately sedated, paralysed if appropriate and monitored throughout the procedure.

A contrast medium may be administered intravenously, to assist in clarifying areas being examined.

The cerebral function analysing monitor (CFAM)

The electroencephalogram, or EEG, is a recording of the electrical activity within the brain. By recording this activity and then analysing it, valuable information can be obtained to assist diagnosis of seizure activity or central nervous system injury/dysfunction.

Different institutions have their own methods of obtaining continuous EEG recordings of the critically ill child. One machine used for this purpose is the CFAM machine and, as it can be the role of nursing staff to set up the machine, attach it to the patient and troubleshoot any mechanical difficulties, the following information may be helpful:

- After the machine has been turned on and set up, ensure that the File Number has been correctly documented, so that the recording can be retrieved if there are problems with the paper print out

- Ensure that symmetry is achieved during placement of electrodes, and that the most appropriate ones are used; caps are available for certain sizes of babies/children

- Careful application – which can mean less is more! – of glue and electrode gel will reduce impedance

- Ensure that both channels – left and right – are shown on the screen

- Impedance should be as low as possible – preferably less than 10 ohms

- More gel may be required to electrodes every few hours to ensure that an effective trace is achieved. If there is a trace from one side of the head only, or the impedance is rising, then check all the electrodes to ensure they are firmly attached and have adequate gel inserted. If the troublesome electrode can be isolated, repositioning it close to its original site may be effective.

As with all monitoring, the EEG trace should be considered along with an overall assessment of the child. Guidelines on its interpretation and significance should be available from the medical staff in the centres where it is used.

FITTING

Fits (seizures) are sudden, abnormal discharges of cerebral neurones (BMJ 1997).

They may be generalised (activity spread through the sub-cortical area, bilateral tonic-clonic activity possibly associated with loss of consciousness), or focal (activity localised in a small area of the cerebral cortex, unilateral tonic-clonic activity).

Tonic phase – rigidity of muscles due to spasm.

Clonic phase – convulsive jerking movements, commonly of limbs and trunk.

Clinical signs of fitting may include the following:

- Changes in:
- blood pressure
- heart rate
- respiratory pattern
- Convulsions
- Cyanosis.

Commonly, specific charts are used to document episodes of fitting, where the following details are recorded:

- Description of the abnormal movements, e.g. smacking lips followed by repeated jerking of right arm
- Duration
- Whether self-resolving or, if medication was required, which drugs were administered and their effect.

It would also be beneficial to record whether the fits were spontaneous or triggered by an intervention, e.g. someone touching or moving the child.

> ⚠ As abnormal movements do not necessarily constitute fits, **write what you see** to prevent inaccurate interpretation.

When an intubated child has been paralysed and sedated, clinical signs of fitting can be masked; the use of EEG monitoring in these circumstances can be valuable.

Causes of fitting

- Structural lesions, e.g.
  - cerebral infarction
  - tumour
  - haematoma
  - abscess
- Infection
  - systemic
  - CNS
  - encephalitis/meningitis
  - high grade pyrexia
- Toxic ingestion
- Metabolic disorders
- Head trauma
- Seizure disorders, e.g. epilepsy
- Hypoxic–ischaemic encephalopathy.

Status epilepticus

This occurs either when a fit lasts for longer than 30 minutes or when successive seizures occur so frequently that the patient does not recover fully between them.

Status epilepticus can be fatal – death may be due to:

- Complications of the convulsion, such as obstruction of the airway or aspiration of vomit
- Overmedication
- Underlying disease process.

Injury to the brain during status epilepticus occurs as a result of one or more of the following:

- Direct injury from repetitive neuronal discharge
- Systemic complications of the convulsions, especially hypoxia from airway obstruction and later acidosis when systemic hypotension occurs
- Underlying disease process.

The most common causes of status epilepticus in children are:

- Febrile status epilepticus
- Sudden reduction in antiepileptic medication
- Acute cerebral trauma
- Idiopathic epilepsy, i.e. cause unknown
- Bacterial meningitis
- Encephalopathy (including Reye's syndrome)
- Poisoning (BMJ 1997).

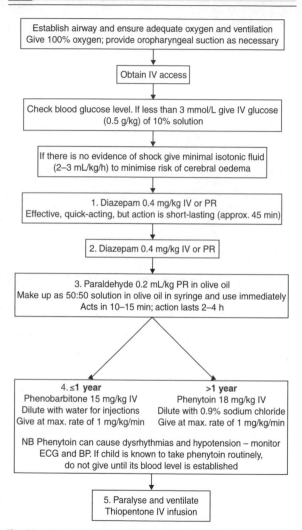

Fig. 6.2 Treatment protocol for status epilepticus (adapted with permission from BMJ 1997)

The treatment protocol for status epilepticus is set out in Figure 6.2. Thiopentone is a general anaesthetic. It is particularly valuable in patients with neurological involvement because of its ability to acutely reduce ICP; it therefore has a cerebroprotective effect (Singer & Webb 1997).

It is an alkaline solution, which will cause irritation if it leaks into subcutaneous tissues – watch for signs of cannula extravasation.

By re-assessing the child after each step of the treatment protocol in Figure 6.2, or guidelines similar to it, the effects of treatment can be evaluated, and the need for further intervention can be decided.

SYNDROME OF INAPPROPRIATE ANTIDIURETIC HORMONE SECRETION (SIADH)

SIADH can develop in any child who sustains injury to or compression of the pituitary or hypothalamus – this may occur as a result of:

- head injury
- intracranial haemorrhage
- encephalopathies (including Guillain-Barré syndrome, meningitis and encephalitis)
- hydrocephalus
- raised ICP
- neurosurgery
- antidiuretic hormone (ADH)-secreting tumours.

ADH or arginine vasopressin is formed in the hypothalamus. It is transported to the posterior pituitary gland, where it is released in response to differences between extracellular and intracellular osmolality. ADH increases the permeability of the renal distal tubule and collecting ducts to water, so that less free water is excreted in the urine, reducing urine volume and increasing concentration. If ADH levels remain elevated, serum hypo-osmolality and hyponatraemia will develop.

Signs and symptoms

Urine volume is often reduced, but the urine osmolality and sodium concentration will be high. If the SIADH continues, water intoxication and hyponatraemic seizures can result from the movement of water from the intravascular space into cerebral tissue.

Management

- Diagnosis is confirmed when patient responds to fluid restriction with correction of hyponatraemia
- Fluids usually restricted to 30–75% maintenance
- If profound hyponatraemia or signs of water intoxication are present (deterioration in level of consciousness or seizures), administration of hypertonic saline (3% sodium chloride) and a diuretic, e.g. frusemide, may be prescribed to increase serum sodium concentration and eliminate excess intravascular water
- Close monitoring of level of consciousness, fluid balance, daily weight, and blood and urine chemistries
- The underlying cause of the SIADH should be treated.

DIABETES INSIPIDUS

Central or neurogenic diabetes insipidus can be observed in children who:

- sustain head injuries
- sustain central nervous system infections
- sustain intraventricular haemorrhages
- undergo neurosurgery.

Neurogenic diabetes insipidus results from decreased production of ADH. When ADH is not synthesised by the hypothalamus, circulating ADH levels are negligible. Renal collecting tubules therefore remain relatively impermeable to water, resulting in insufficient reabsorption. Large amounts of water are lost in urine. Intravascular volume is quickly depleted, and haemoconcentration produces hypernatraemia. The osmotic gradient causes fluid to shift from the intracellular to the intravascular space and that fluid is quickly lost from the circulation. Intravascular hypovolaemia stimulates aldosterone secretion, leading to the reabsorption of water and sodium from the proximal renal tubule. If the child's fluid intake is limited to intravenous therapy, and s/he is not able to drink freely, unrecognised diabetes insipidus can quickly produce hypovolaemia, hypernatraemia and serum hyperosmolality.

Signs and symptoms

- Polyuria – the excretion of large amounts of very dilute urine with low osmolality, low sodium concentration and very low specific gravity – important to detect this condition early because the critically ill child can become hypovolaemic and hypernatraemic very quickly

• Irritability, tachycardia, low CVP, weak peripheral pulses and hypotension, metabolic acidosis, prolonged capillary refill time

• In infant, anterior fontanelle depressed

• Reduced body weight.

Management

• Rapid replacement of urinary fluid and electrolyte losses and provision of ADH in the form of a drug

• Close monitoring of fluid balance, intravascular volume, systemic perfusion and electrolyte balance

• Positive response to vasopressin will be seen by decrease in urine volume to approximately 1 mL/kg/h, a rise in urine specific gravity to more than 1.010 and osmolality to 280–300 mmol/L (Hazinski 1992)

• By calculating fluid replacement on hourly urine output, it is easier to taper this in response to vasopressin.

GUILLAIN–BARRÉ SYNDROME

Guillain–Barré syndrome is the association of a preceding infection, progressive motor weakness and elevated CSF protein content. The preceding illness may be upper respiratory infection or viral illness. It most commonly occurs in children aged 4–10 years, although it can occur in any age group. The cause is unknown but appears to be related to an autoimmune or inflammatory processes that produce inflammation of nerves and nerve roots.

• The inflammation of the nerves and nerve roots involves the endodural and epidural blood vessels

• First the myelin becomes oedematous; demyelination develops, producing decreased speed and intensity of peripheral nerve conduction. Nerve degeneration may also occur.

Signs and symptoms

• Child may complain of tingling/numbness/pain in fingers and toes, and soon demonstrates weakness of the lower extremities and possible loss of deep tendon reflexes

• Over a period of several days or weeks, motor weakness ascends to include arms and possibly the cranial nerves. If the

intercostal muscles are paralysed the child will require ventilatory assistance

• Glossopharyngeal and vagus nerve dysfunction may develop
and produce impairment of the gag and swallow reflexes

• During the initial stages of the illness, autonomic instability
may be evident, demonstrated by wide fluctuations in blood
pressure, cardiac arrhythmias, diaphoresis (excessive sweat-
ing) and pupil dilation and constriction.

Recovery from Guillain–Barré syndrome usually begins
approximately 4 weeks after the onset of symptoms. Although
the majority of children make a complete recovery, a small
number of affected patients die, some demonstrate significant
neurological disorders and others may be prone to relapses.

Management

This is largely supportive, with weaning gradually taking
place as the child recovers:

• Thorough and frequent neurological assessment, including
limb strength and movement, and cranial nerve function

• Ventilation in order to protect airway as well as to assist
child's own respiratory effort

• Careful monitoring of cardiovascular function, with treatment of arrhythmias and hypotension that result in a compro-
mise of systemic perfusion

• Provision of adequate calorific intake (either enterally or
parenterally)

• Physiotherapy and maintenance of skin integrity

• Psychological aspects of care – the child may be hospit-
alised for a considerable length of time, and is likely to be
frightened, as well as depressed, by the disease process; continuity of care, consideration of family involvement, play specialist, position of child's bed in a busy PICU are all important

• Support of family and child through the critical period of
an illness from which the child may well recover but which
may prove extremely frightening, with consistent information and caregivers (adapted from Hazinski 1992).

MENINGITIS

Meningitis is an acute inflammation of the meninges and
cerebrospinal fluid, which occurs more commonly in children
than adults, particularly in children between 1 month and

5 years of age. It is most commonly caused by bacteria, although it can also be caused by viruses. The most important causes of bacterial meningitis in children are *Haemophilus influenzae* and *Neisseria meningitidis*. Other organisms include *Streptococcus pneumoniae* and *Staphylococcus*.

Immunisation against *Haemophilus influenzae* type B is now routine, via the Hib vaccine, given with the triple DPT vaccine at the ages of 2, 3 and 4 months. These forms of meningitis usually result from the extension of a localised infection, with transient bacteraemia and central nervous system spread of the organism.

Signs and symptoms

- Difficult to assess in infants: extreme irritability, with high pitched 'cerebral cry' or lethargy with vomiting and fever
- If intracranial pressure is high, anterior fontanelle may be full and tense
- Child may complain of headache and photophobia (extreme sensitivity to light)
- Neck stiffness
- Kernig's sign (pain associated with extension of the knee when the thighs are flexed)
- Brudzinski's sign (flexion of neck stimulates flexion at knees and hips)
- Purpuric skin rash – small dark red spots (petechiae) caused by capillaries bleeding into the skin indicates meningococcal disease.

The importance of early recognition of symptoms so that effective treatment can be commenced as soon as possible cannot be over emphasised.

Management

- Full blood screen for analysis will be performed, including blood cultures
- Lumbar puncture to obtain cerebrospinal fluid (CSF) specimen may be performed UNLESS the child is believed to have raised ICP, when it would be omitted
- If meningitis is suspected, while awaiting the results of specimens taken, the administration of IV antibiotics will commence – centres have their own protocols, but cefotaxime and ceftriaxone are popular
- It is now common practice in many PICUs for children with meningitis to be nursed on an open unit, rather than in a

cubicle, once the first dose of IV antibiotics has been given –
refer to local infection control policy

• Once the causative agent has been identified, the appropriate antibiotics will be prescribed

• Full neurological assessment in conjunction with holistic assessment

• Intubation and ventilation may be necessary to maintain a patent airway and to treat raised ICP

• Fluid restriction will be required according to local policy

• If the child shows signs of sepsis (e.g. deranged clotting, hypotension (late sign), poor capillary refill time and toe–core gap) that do not respond to boluses of fluid, inotropic support may need to be commenced.

NB Provision of prophylactic oral antibiotics to family members and others who have had recent, prolonged, close contact with the child, is common. Examples of these are ciprofloxacin or rifampicin. When rifampicin is administered, to avoid alarm, those taking it need to be informed that it turns bodily secretions, e.g. urine, red. If rifampicin is administered to women of childbearing age, it is important to inform them that this drug obliterates the action of the contraceptive pill.

Meningitis is a notifiable disease – the medical staff will have to therefore notify the Public Health Inspector of the occurrence.

Viral meningitis may require only supportive care, as this form is usually much milder than bacterial meningitis.

Table 6.1 The cranial nerves (adapted with permission from McCance & Heuther 1992)		
Cranial nerve	**Function**	**Assessment**
I Olfactory	Smell	Difficult to assess accurately in small children.
II Optic	Vision	Assess ability to see objects near and far, object moving into visual field from periphery and identifying colours.
III Oculomotor	Pupil constriction, movement of eye and eyelid	Pupils should constrict when light is applied to each; consensual constriction (constriction in response to light directed to other eye) should be observed; eye should follow moving object; eyelids should

		raise equally when eyes are open. Ptosis (drooping eyelid) and lateral downward deviation of eye with pupil dilatation + decreased response to light = oculomotor injury.
IV Trochlear	Movement of eye, (superior oblique muscle)	Assess ability of eyes to track object down through visual field – damage stops eyes moving downwards + medially. Diplopia (blurred or double vision) may be present.
V Trigeminal	Sensation to most of face + movement of jaw	Cover eyes; sharp/soft to skin + assess sensation. Check clench + move jaw + chew.
VI Abducens	Lateral movement of eye	Assess eye movement in socket tracking object – when object close to child, both eyes should track it + move together. Child may turn head towards weakened muscle to prevent diplopia.
VII Facial	Motor innervation of face, sensation to anterior tongue + tears	Ask child to make faces (demonstrate) + assess symmetry of face. Tears should be produced when crying. Drops of sugar/salt on tongue – test taste.
VIII Vestibulocochlear (hearing)	Hearing + equilibrium	Clap hands – startle reflex in infants; blink reflex to sudden sound. NB Cranial nerves III and IV must be intact for normal response to following: *'Dolls eyes' manoeuvre (oculocephalic reflex)*: As child's head is turned, eyes should shift in sockets in direction OPPOSITE to head rotation; this constitutes the normal response. *Cold water calorics (oculovestibular reflex)*: Normally, instillation of cold water into ear should produce lateral nystagmus (rapid involuntary movement of the eyes – up and down/side to side/rotating); not to be performed if child is conscious. These tests are typically performed as part of brain stem testing.

Cranial nerve	Function	Assessment
IX Glossopharyngeal	Motor fibres to throat + voluntary muscles of swallowing + speech	Evaluate swallow, cough + gag (tests IX + X together). If possible assess clarity of speech.
X Vagus	Sensory + motor impulses for pharynx	Test as above – particularly cough + gag.
XI Spinal accessory	Major innervation of sternoclei-domastoid + upper trapezius	Ask child to shrug shoulders and assess contraction of trapezius muscles; child to turn head as sternocleidomastoid muscle is palpated (long muscle in neck – serves to rotate head + flex neck).
XII Hypoglossal	Innervation of the tongue	Ask child to stick out tongue. Squeeze nose of infant – mouth should open + tip of tongue should rise in mouth.

Many rhymes have been devised to help remember the cranial nerves. Here is an example:

On
Old
Olympus
Towering
Top
A
Finn
And   Acoustic (vestibulochlear)
German
Viewed
Some
Hops

REFERENCES

Allen D 1993 Ventriculostomy. Surg Nurse July: 17–20
Birdsall C, Grief L 1990 How do you manage extraventricular drainage? Am J Nurs November: 47–49
BMJ 1997 Advanced paediatric life support – the practical approach, 2nd edn. British Medical Journal, London

Evans O B 1987 Manual of child neurology. Churchill Livingstone, New York

Feldman Z, Kanter M, Robertson C et al 1992 Effect of head elevation on intracranial pressure and cerebral blood flow in head injured patients. J Neurosurg 76: 207–211

Fisher M D 1997 Pediatric traumatic brain injury. Crit Care Nurs Q 20(1): 36–51

Germon K 1994 Intracranial pressure monitoring in the 1990s. Crit Care Nurs Q 17(1): 21–23

Hazinski M F (ed) 1992 Nursing care of the critically ill child, 2nd edn. C V Mosby, St Louis, MO

Kerr M, Brucia J 1993 Hyperventilation in the head injured patient: an effective treatment modality? Heart and Lung 22: 516–521

Lower J 1992 Rapid neuro assessment. Am J Nurs June: 38–45

McCance K L, Heuther S 1992 In: Hazinski M F (ed) Nursing care of the critically ill child, 2nd edn. C V Mosby, St Louis, MO

Schinner K, Chisholm A, Grap M, Siva P, Hallinan M, LaVoice-Hawkins A 1995 The effects of auditory stimuli on intracranial pressure and cerebral perfusion pressure in traumatic brain injury. J Neurosci Nurs 27(6): 348–354

Shann F 1996 Drug doses, 9th edn. Collective Pty, Melbourne, Victoria

Shiozaki T, Sugimoto H, Taneda M et al 1998 Selection of severely head injured patients for mild hypothermia therapy. J Neurosurg 89: 206–211

Simpson D, Reilly P 1982 Paediatric coma scale. Lancet 2: 450

Singer M, Webb A 1997 Oxford handbook of critical care. Oxford University Press, Oxford

Singh N C (ed) 1997 Manual of pediatric critical care. W B Saunders, Philadelphia, PA

Teasdale G, Jennett B 1974 Assessment of coma and impaired consciousness, a practical scale. Lancet 2: 81–84

FURTHER READING

Chitnavis B P, Polkey C E 1998 ICP monitoring. Care Crit Ill 14(3): 80–84

Reynolds E A 1992 Controversies in caring for the child with a head injury. Man Clin Nurs September/October: 246–251

7

FLUIDS AND NUTRITION

When children are admitted to hospital, it is important to get an accurate weight, as fluids and medications are often based upon this. If the child presents in a critical condition then weighing the child would obviously be inappropriate; Table 7.1 therefore gives mean weights of babies and children on the 50th centile, which can be used as a guide, or an estimation can be calculated using the following formula.

Estimated body weight in a child aged 1–10 years of age:

$$\text{Weight (kg)} = (\text{Age in years} + 4) \times 2.$$

Table 7.1 A guide to weight: mean weight of babies and children on 50th centile (adapted from Department of Health 1991. Crown copyright material is reproduced with the permission of the Controller of Her Majesty's Stationery Office)

Age	Mean weight (kg)
3 months	5.9
6 months	7.7
9 months	8.8
1 year	9.7
2 years	12
4 years	15.9
7.5 years	24
10.5 years	32.8
12.5 years	40
15.5 years	54.5

Table 7.2 is a guide to fluid requirements per 24 hours according to the age of the infant or child.

The daily fluid requirement chart serves as guidance only, as fluid requirements may be increased or decreased in certain circumstances:

- Increased fluids may be required in patients with a pyrexia, with burns requiring radiant heat, undergoing phototherapy or to replace lost volume
- Decreased fluids may be required in patients following cardiac surgery, or patients in renal or heart failure.

Table 7.2 Daily fluid maintenance requirement in babies and children based on age	
Age	**Fluid requirement (mL/kg/24h) – up to:**
0–3 months	150
4–6 months	130
7–9 months	120
10–12 months	110
1–3 years	95
4–6 years	85
7–10 years	75
11–14 years	55
15–18 years	50

Table 7.3 Estimated average daily energy requirement by age (from Department of Health 1991. Crown copyright material is reproduced with the permission of the Controller of Her Majesty's Stationery Office)	
Age	**Kilocalories/24 h**
0–3 months	515–545
4–6 months	645–690
7–9 months	765–825
10–12 months	865–920
1–3 years	1165–1230
4–6 years	1545–1715
7–10 years	1740–1970
11–14 years	1845–2220
15–18 years	2110–2755

The lower end of the range refers to females and the upper end refers to males

Table 7.3 shows recommended daily energy requirements for healthy infants and children which will alter if the child becomes unwell or suffers trauma.

ENTERAL FEEDING

When infants or children are admitted to paediatric intensive care, enteral feeding is commenced whenever possible. Many units have developed practice guidelines to facilitate establishment of full enteral feeding within specified time limits and an example of this is given in Figure 7.1. It may be necessary to give parenteral nutrition alongside enteral

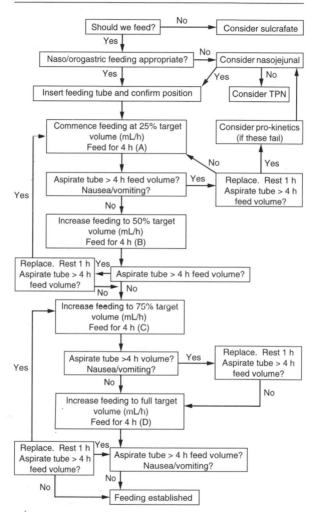

Fig. 7.1 Paediatric Intensive Care Unit enteral feeding guidelines (reproduced with permission from Martin and Cox 1998)

nutrition if absorption is poor or insufficient calories are being given.

The time taken to establish full enteral feeds through the normal absorption pathway of A, B, C and D takes 16 hours. Section C, however, is optional and can be omitted if required, and the time taken to establish full feeds is then 12 hours.

Enteral feeding practice guidelines (Martin & Cox 1998)

Nasogastric tube:

- Mark the nasogastric tube at nasal exit site in order to detect slippage (Fawcett 1995)
- Confirm nasogastric tube placement using pH paper or X-ray (Metheny 1988)
- If unable to obtain a sample from the gut, try changing the child's position or flushing the tube with sterile water and withdrawing (Metheny 1988)
- Air insufflation to check nasogastric position is not recommended (Metheny 1988)
- Change PVC nasogastric tubes every 3–4 days according to manufacturers' instructions
- Consider fine-bore (silicone) tubes for long-term nasogastric feeding (Briggs 1996).

Suitable feeds:

- Consult paediatric dietician's written recommendations regarding suitable feeds or calorie supplements.

Tolerance:

- Nurse child in an upright position wherever possible to minimise reflux (Fawcett 1995)
- Consider constipation as a cause of large aspirates, nausea, vomiting and/or diarrhoea.

Aspirates:

- Volumes above 200 mL may indicate intolerance in older children (McClave et al 1992)
- A single high-volume aspirate does not constitute intolerance (McClave et al 1992)
- Assess aspirates (? predigested milk or ? bile). Replace all aspirates wherever possible. Discuss persistent high-volume aspirates with members of the multidisciplinary team
- Fluid-replace discarded volumes as indicated in order to maintain pH and electrolyte balance (Hazinski 1992)

- If unable to progress to full feeds, consider alternative ways of supplementing nutritional requirements.

Nausea and vomiting:

- Rest the gut for short periods as indicated (Taylor 1989)
- If persistent, consider changing the feed, introducing pro-kinetics, e.g. cisapride, or feeding via the nasojejunal route (Taylor 1989).

Diarrhoea:

- Review medication (Edes et al 1990)
- Send stool sample to microbiology for culture and sensitivity and testing for *Clostridium difficile* (Edes et al 1990)
- Discuss with dietitian
- Consider changing the feed or adding fibre (Heimburger 1990)
- If no other cause is found, consider stopping the feed for 24 hours to exclude feed as cause (Edes et al 1990).

Infection control:

- Milk feeds should not hang for more than 4 h (Anderton 1995)
- Disposable feed administration sets should be changed every 24 h (Kohn 1991, Patchell et al 1998) – label and date the set
- Prepacked feeds once opened should be stored 4°C or less for a maximum of 24 h (Anderton 1995) – label and date the feeds
- Aprons and non-sterile gloves should be worn when handling feeds or administration sets (Anderton 1995)
- Disposable administration sets should be primed on a 'clean' surface
- Bottles, cans, cartons and the access port on the administration set should be alcowiped prior to use (Anderton 1995)
- Feeds should be decanted using a non-touch technique
- The designated port on the administration set should be used for nasogastric aspiration and the administration of medication
- Nasogastric tubes should be flushed with sterile water after the administration of medication. Feeding systems should be handled only as much as is absolutely necessary (Anderton 1995).

Continuous feeding regime:

- All children being fed continuously should receive a break equivalent to 4 h total
- The feeding regime should be determined according to the individual
- Rest periods should be determined according to the maintenance of blood glucose, medication administration and proposed medical intervention.

TYPES OF FEEDING AND PRODUCTS AVAILABLE

It is widely accepted that breast-feeding is the optimum mode of feeding for a baby during the first few months of life. There are, however, many products available to give a baby who for whatever reason cannot be breast-fed. Suitable products appropriate to age and weight are discussed below for children in hospital who are unable to eat normally.

Infant milks and children's feed

Use of milk products and children's feeds
- Under 6 months of age use baby milk formula as preferred
- 6–12 months use formula as previous or follow-on formula
- Over 1 year use follow-on formula, full-fat cows' milk or standard child formula, e.g. Nutrini (1 kcal/mL), Nutrini Extra (1.5 kcal/mL)
- Above 6 years use children's feed, e.g. Fresubin, Ensure Plus.

Premature babies
Preterm babies with birthweight below 1.8 kg:

- SMA low birthweight formula, Osterprem, Prematil, Nutriprem.

Preterm babies above 2 kg until 6 months of age:

- Premcare, Nutriprem 2.

Full-term babies
Whey based milks:

- SMA Gold, Cow & Gate Premium, Farleys First, Aptamil.

Casein based milks:

- SMA White, Cow & Gate Plus, Farleys Second, Milumil.

Follow-on formulas – usually used from 6 months onwards:

- SMA Progress, Cow & Gate Step Up, Farleys Follow On, Milupa Forward, Boots Milk Drink.

Soya milk (for milk protein intolerance):

- Infasoy, Wysoy, Ostersoy, Prosobee, Isomil.

Protein hydrolysates – (for malabsorption):

- Nutramigen, Pregestimil, Prejomin, Pepti Junior, Peptide 0–2, MCT Peptide 0–2, Alfare.

Elemental (amino acid feed):

- Neocate, Elemental.

Other products (for use in patients with chylothorax or liver disease):

- Monogen (93% MCT), Portagen, Caprilon (70% MCT).

Children's feeds
- Nutrini Standard or Extra, Frebini, Paediasure, Paediasure Fibre.

Supplements include:

- *Calories* – Maxijul, Duocal, Calogen
- *Protein* – Maxipro, Vitapro.

All formula milks in the UK are gluten free (Shaw & Lawson 1994).

SPECIAL DIETS FOR SPECIAL KIDS

Infants and children with certain inborn errors of metabolism often have specific dietary requirements. General principles of dietary needs are highlighted; they are only intended as a guide to give nurses some ideas of general requirements and will not replace specialist advice from dietetic services.

Coeliac disease

- Coeliac disease is a malabsorption syndrome where the proximal intestinal mucosa lose their villous structure and the absorptive function becomes impaired

- It is precipitated by the ingestion of gluten in foods and symptoms usually start appearing in children several months after the introduction of solids containing gluten
- A gluten-free diet is required and supplements of vitamins may be given.

Cystic fibrosis

- Cystic fibrosis is a hereditary disorder with widespread dysfunction of exocrine glands, characterised by chronic pulmonary disease, pancreatic deficiency, abnormally high levels of electrolytes in the sweat and occasionally biliary cirrhosis
- Many patients will require pancreatic enzyme replacement therapy
- A high-protein, high-energy diet is required with added vitamins and trace elements.

Diabetes mellitus

- Diabetes mellitus is a metabolic disorder where the pancreas becomes unable to maintain normal insulin production, causing hyperglycaemia, glycosuria and polyuria
- In children this is frequently controlled by a combination of diet and insulin
- A well-balanced diet is required with minimal refined sugars, free fructose and an even distribution of carbohydrate throughout the day.

Inborn errors of metabolism

This may be divided into disorders of amino acid metabolism, organic acidaemias and urea cycle defects. Details of each condition should be sought as only a brief outline will be given of a few disorders.

Phenylketonuria

- Phenylketonuria is a disorder of amino acid metabolism
- It is characterised by a deficiency of the liver enzyme phenylalanine hydroxylase, which is needed to breakdown the amino acid phenylalanine to tyrosine
- This disorder will be detected by the Guthrie test (a simple blood test taken once the infant is established on milk feeds and usually performed at around 1 week of age)

- Phenylalanine is essential for growth so once the initially high level of phenylalanine has been reduced by a phenylalanine-free diet, it is gradually reintroduced at a low level
- A diet low in phenylalanine with supplements of amino acids, vitamins and trace elements will be required to an age of around 6–8 years when the nervous system is less vulnerable to elevated levels of phenylalanine and compliance falls (Hull & Johnston 1996).

Maple syrup urine disease

- Maple syrup urine disease is caused by a deficiency of branched chain 2 ketoacid dehydrogenase enzyme complex, which results in the accumulation of three essential amino acids – leucine, isoleucine and valine
- The infant presents in the first few days of life with toxic encephalopathy and the characteristic urine that smells of maple syrup
- A low-protein diet (particularly low leucine) is required with supplements of amino acids, vitamins and minerals
- If the child becomes unwell, a protein-free, high-energy diet is required (Francis 1987).

Organic acidaemias

- There are several other organic acidaemias, all due to different malfunctioning or absent enzymes that involve different amino acids
- The basic principles of dietary management include a low-protein diet and supplements of vitamins, minerals and trace elements; energy supplements are also required
- During periods of illness, the patient is at risk of developing metabolic acidosis due to accumulation of organic acids, so protein intake is usually withdrawn for a few days and an emergency diet, predominantly of a glucose polymer, or even total parenteral nutrition is given (Contact a Family 1997, Shaw & Lawson 1994)
- Supplements of carnitine or other amino acid derivatives may be required.

Urea cycle defects

- Deficiencies of specific enzymes cause disorders in the urea cycle and lead to a buildup of ammonia in the blood and cerebrospinal fluid
- The infant or child may present with neurological abnormalities due to toxic levels of ammonia

- A low-protein diet is required to try to keep ammonia levels as low as possible, plus supplements of arginine (sodium benzoate, phenylacetate and citrulline may also be prescribed)
- In illness, the emergency regime of no protein and a high-calorie diet may be imposed.

Glycogen storage diseases

Glucose-6-phosphatase deficiency

- This is an enzyme deficiency of glucose-6-phosphatase, which disrupts normal maintenance of plasma glucose levels
- It usually presents in infancy with hepatomegaly, hypoglycaemia and metabolic acidosis
- Frequent glucose/carbohydrate feeds are required to prevent hypoglycaemia
- Avoid fructose and galactose in the diet as they cannot be converted to glycogen and will be metabolised to lactate.

Galactosaemia

- Galactosaemia is an inborn error of galactose metabolism as a result of enzyme deficiency
- The majority of infants present in first week of life with jaundice, failure to thrive, vomiting and hepato-megaly, as breast milk and most infant formulas contain galactose
- Galactose must be eliminated from the diet as far as possible for life.

TOTAL PARENTERAL NUTRITION

Total parenteral nutrition (TPN) consists of sterile solutions that are made up in pharmacy and are administered directly into the blood stream via a vein. The solutions:

- are made up of amino acids, carbohydrates and lipids
- should be protected from light to prevent the formation of free radicals
- should be stored in a fridge until used
- should be administered via a central line, especially if the glucose concentration is greater than 12.5%, and on a unique line saved for the sole use of TPN

Table 7.4 How to prepare 7.5%, 12.5% and 15% dextrose solutions (reproduced with permission from R Urquhart, personal communication, 1998)

Concentration required (%)	Quantity of 50% dextrose (mL)	Add to 500 mL of dextrose
7.5	31.1	5%
12.5	33.3	10%
15	71.3	10%

- should be double-checked against the prescription before administration
- should be changed using aseptic precautions.

Patients on TPN should have daily weight, urine glucose and electrolytes, urea and electrolytes, full blood count, fluid balance and initially 6-hourly blood glucose tested. Every fortnight measure plasma chemistry for copper, manganese, selenium and zinc (adapted from Guy's, St Thomas' and Lewisham Hospitals 1999).

SALINE AND DEXTROSE SOLUTION

- 4% & 0.18% dextrose saline solution contains 4 g of dextrose and 30 mmol of sodium and chloride per 100 mL
- 5% dextrose contains 5 g dextrose/100 mL
- 10% dextrose contains 10 g dextrose/100 mL
- 50% dextrose contains 50 g dextrose/100 mL.

On occasion it is necessary to make up solutions of dextrose that are not available as standard commercially prepared products (Table 7.4).

INSENSIBLE LOSS

This occurs mostly through the skin and the respiratory tract and accounts for approximately 30 mL/kg/24 h. However, fever will increase insensible loss by 12% per 1°C rise in temperature above 37.2°C (Shann 1996).

BURNS

See Chapter 9 for estimation of percentage burns and fluid replacement regimes.

REFERENCES

Anderton A 1995 Reducing bacterial contamination in enteral tube feeds. Br J Nurs 4(7): 368–376

Briggs D 1996 What type of naso-gastric tube should we use in the intensive care unit? Intens Crit Care Nurs 12: 102–105

Contact a Family 1997 Organic acidaemias UK: a leaflet for parents and teachers. Contact a Family, London

Department of Health 1991 Dietary reference values for food energy and nutrients for the United Kingdom. HMSO, London: p xix.

Edes T E et al 1990 Diarrhoea in tube fed patients: feeding formula not necessarily the cause. Am J Med 88: 91–93

Fawcett H 1995 Nutritional support for hospital patients. Nurs Stand 9(48): 25–28

Francis D 1987 Diets for sick children, 4th edn. Blackwell, Oxford

Guy's, St Thomas' and Lewisham Hospitals 1999 Paediatric formulary 4th edn. Guy's, St Thomas' and Lewisham Hospitals, London

Hazinski M F(ed) 1992 Nursing care of the critically ill child, 2nd edn. C V Mosby, St Louis, MO

Heimburger D C 1990 Diarrhoea with enteral feeding: will the real cause stand up please? Am J Med 88: 89–90

Hull D, Johnston D I 1996 Essential paediatrics, 3rd edn. Churchill Livingstone, Edinburgh

Kohn C L 1991 The relationship between enteral formula contamination and length of delivery set usage. J Parent Enteral Nutrit 15(5): 567–571

McClave S A et al 1992 Use of residual volume as a marker for enteral feeding intolerance: prospective blinded comparison with physical examination and radiographic findings. J Parent Enteral Nutrit 16(2): 99–105

Martin L, Cox S 1998 Paediatric intensive care enteral feeding guideline and practice guidelines. Unpublished.

Metheny N 1988 Measures to test placement of naso-gastric and naso-intestinal tubes: a review. Nurs Res 37(6): 324–329

Patchell C J et al 1998 Reducing bacterial contamination of enteral feeds. Arch Dis Child 78: 166–168

Shann F 1996 Drug doses, 9th edn. Collective Pty Ltd

Shaw V, Lawson M 1994 Clinical paediatric dietetics 1st edn. Blackwell, Oxford

Taylor S 1989 Preventing complications in enteral feeding. Prof Nurse Feb: 247–249

FURTHER READING

McClaren D S, Burman D 1982 Textbook of paediatric nutrition, 2nd edn. Churchill Livingstone, Edinburgh

Taitz L S, Wardley B 1989 Handbook of child nutrition. Oxford University Press, Oxford

BLOOD AND ELECTROLYTES: NORMAL VALUES AND TRANSFUSION

8

This chapter highlights normal blood values, general information about blood products, storage and administration and a guide to common electrolyte imbalance, outlining causes, diagnosis and principles of treatment. Consult local policies and suppliers for further information. The normal ranges of blood values given are intended as a guide and may vary in different hospitals.

NORMAL VALUES: FULL BLOOD COUNT, CLOTTING, UREA AND ELECTROLYTES

Table 8.1 Full blood count for normal infants and children (reproduced with permission from Dacie & Lewis 1997)

Age	Units	Newborn full-term	Up to 6 months	2–6 years	6–12 years
Red blood cells (RBC)	$\times 10^{12}$/L	6.0 ± 1.0	3.8 ± 0.8	4.6 ± 0.7	4.6 ± 0.6
Haemoglobin (Hb)	g/dL	16.5 ± 3.0	11.5 ± 2.0	12.5 ± 1.5	13.5 ± 2.0
Packed cell volume (PCV)	L/L	0.54 ± 0.10	0.35 ± 0.07	0.37 ± 0.03	0.40 ± 0.05
Mean corpuscular volume (MCV)	fl	110 ± 10	91 ± 17	81 ± 6	86 ± 8
Mean corpuscular haemoglobin (MCH)	pg	34 ± 3	30 ± 5	27 ± 3	29 ± 4
Platelets	$\times 10^9$/L	150–400	150–400	150–400	150–400
White blood count (WBC)	$\times 10^9$/L	18 ± 8	12 ± 6	10 ± 5	9 ± 4
Neutrophils	$\times 10^9$/L	5.0–13.0	1.5–9.0	1.5–8.0	2.0–8.0
Lymphocytes	$\times 10^9$/L	3.0–10.0	4.0–10.0	6.0–9.0	1.0–5.0
Monocytes	$\times 10^9$/L	0.7–1.5	0.1–1.0	0.1–1.0	0.1–1.0
Eosinophils	$\times 10^9$/L	0.2–1.0	0.2–1.0	0.2–1.0	0.1–1.0
Reticulocytes	$\times 10^9$/L	200–500	40–100	20–200	20–200

CLOTTING VALUES

Table 8.2 Clotting values			
	Abbreviation	Value	Standard units
Prothrombin time	PT	11–16	seconds
International normalised ratio	INR	0.8–1.1	Ratio
Activated PT	APTT	0.8–1.2	Ratio
Fibrinogen		2.02–4.24	g/L

UREA AND ELECTROLYTES

Table 8.3 Urea and electrolytes		
	Value	Standard units
Sodium	135–145	mmol/L
Potassium	3.5–5.0	mmol/L
Chloride	98–107	mmol/L
Bicarbonate	22–32	mmol/L
Anion gap	7–17	mmol/L
Urea	2.5–7.5	mmol/L
Creatinine	40–90	µmol/L
Calcium	2.19–2.51	mmol/L
Alb. corrected calcium	2.19–2.51	mmol/L
Magnesium	0.65–0.95	mmol/L
Phosphate	1.2–1.8	mmol/L
Total protein	62–81	g/L
Albumin	37–56	g/L
Alkaline phosphatase	145–320	U/L
Total bilirubin	0–22	µmol/L
Alanine transaminase	0–55	U/L
Aspartate transaminase	0–35	U/L
Gamma glutamyl transpeptidase	8–78	U/L
C reactive protein	<7	mg/L

NORMAL BLOOD VOLUMES

- *Preterm babies*: approximately 100 mL/kg
- *Infants*: approximately 80 mL/kg
- *Children*: approximately 70 mL/kg.

TRANSFUSION COMPATIBILITY

Blood should be cross-matched before the patient is transfused wherever possible but in emergency situations blood group O Rh D negative is sometimes used.

Table 8.4 Transfusion compatibility for ABO group and Rhesus factor (adapted with permission from Shann 1996)

	Whole blood	Platelets	Fresh frozen plasma	Cryoprecipitate	Human albumin solution
Blood group O	O	O	Any	O	Any
Blood group A	A or O	A or O	A or AB	A	Any
Blood group B	B or O	B or O	B or AB	A*	Any
Blood group AB	Any	Any	AB	A*	Any
Rhesus compatibility	Rhesus compatibility required	Not required, except Rh D –ve females require Rh D –ve	Preferable, especially Rh D –ve females	Preferable – especially Rh D –ve females	Not applicable
Special giving set/ filter required	Blood giving set	Platelet giving set	Blood giving set	Blood or platelet giving set	15 μm filter (see manufacturers' instructions)

* Many transfusion centres only produce Group O or A cryoprecipitate.

GELOFUSINE AND TRANSFUSION PRODUCTS

Gelofusine

This is a sterile modified fluid gelatin in saline, a colloidal plasma volume substitute. Gelofusine can increase blood volume, cardiac output, stroke volume, blood pressure, urine output and oxygen delivery.

Half-life: around 4 h – the majority of the dose is eliminated by renal excretion within 24 h.

4.5% human albumin solution

This is used for volume replacement of plasma, e.g. in clinical management of hypovolaemic shock or burns. The only benefit over other colloidal solutions is a longer half-life but it is much more expensive.

Half-life: around 19 days in a healthy adult (no information regarding half-life in children).

The use of human albumin solution is currently under review. Consult local policy for use.

Whole blood, red cells, red cells with additives

Whole blood or packed cells are transfused where major blood loss has occurred, for haemoglobinopathies and in patients with severe anaemias.

Calculation to determine amount of blood required for transfusion

Amount of packed cells required (mL) = weight (kg) × 3 × desired rise in Hb (g/dL).

Once plasma has been removed from whole blood, additives are used to re-suspend red cells and these are designed to maintain the red cells in optimum condition during storage.

Red cells CPDA = added citrate, phosphate, dextrose and adenine.

Red cells SAGM = added sodium chloride, adenine, glucose and mannitol.

Irradiated blood is used in immunocompromised patients and those with depressed T-cell immunity.

Cytomegalovirus (CMV)-negative blood should be used for all neonatal transfusions, as infection caused by Cytomegalovirus can result in neurological deficits (Halliday et al 1985).

CMV is leukocyte-associated; therefore leukocyte filtered cellular components will reduce the risk of CMV transmission.

Fresh frozen plasma

Fresh frozen plasma is often used following cardiopulmonary bypass to help correct prolonged clotting times and improve haemostasis, or may be used where there is evidence of microvascular bleeding and abnormal coagulation.

This occasionally causes severe anaphylactic reactions, especially if infused rapidly.

Dosage is dependent on the clinical condition of the patient, but 12–15 mL/kg is a common dose.

Fresh frozen plasma has not been shown to transmit CMV (McClelland 1996).

Half-life: around 4 days in the circulation.

> ⚠️ Measure the clinical response, prothrombin time (PT) and partial prothromboplastin time (PTT).

Platelets

Platelets may be given where severe microvascular bleeding occurs, e.g. in disseminated intravascular coagulation (DIC).

These should preferably be ABO- and Rh D-compatible as a transfusion could contain enough volume of plasma from a single donor to cause a risk of haemolysis if the donor has potent cell antibodies.

Platelet infusion occasionally results in severe anaphylactic reaction, especially if infused too quickly.

Half-life: 5 days in circulation.

Dose: dependent on clinical condition, usually around 10 mL/kg

Cryoprecipitate

Cryoprecipitate will be given to increase the fibrinogen level, e.g. in a patient who has developed DIC.

This is obtained by allowing the frozen plasma from a single donation to thaw at 4°C and removing the supernatant. It is rich in factor VIII, von Willebrand's factor and fibrinogen. Cryoprecipitate has not been shown to transmit CMV (McClelland 1996).

This occasionally can cause severe anaphylactic reactions if infused rapidly.

Dose: usually 10 mL/kg

Do not add any drugs or additives to blood products received (e.g. calcium can cause citrated blood to clot, 5% dextrose can lyse red cells).

Red cell products

Added chemicals are used to re-suspend packed red cells after plasma has been removed (Table 8.5). They are designed to maintain the cells in good condition during storage.

Table 8.5 Red cell products and additives (McClelland 1996. Crown copyright material is reproduced with the permission of the Controller of Her Majesty's Stationery Office)

	Added chemicals	Points to note
Red cells	Citrate, phosphate, dextrose adenine (CPDA)	
Red cells – additive solution	Sodium chloride, adenine, mannitol, glucose (SAGM)	Not recommended for exchange or large-volume transfusion of neonates
Red cells – buffy coat removed	CPDA or SAGM	May reduce the risk of non-haemolytic febrile transfusion reactions in patients who have reacted previously to transfusion
Red cells – leukocyte depleted	CPDA or SAGM	Can help reduce the development of allo-antibodies to leukocyte antigens – an alternative to CMV-negative product; should **not** be used to avoid risk of graft-versus-host disease: for this indication, irradiated components **must** be used
Whole blood	CPDA	The large volume of plasma increases risk of hypervolaemia and cardiac failure in susceptible patients

Blood components

It is important to follow local policies and protocols when ordering and administering blood products. Table 8.6 provides guidelines regarding storage, shelf life and recommended transfusion times.

Table 8.6 Blood components – storage and administration (adapted from McClelland 1996. Crown copyright material is reproduced with the permission of the Controller of her Majesty's Stationery Office)

	Storage temperature	Shelf life	Longest time from leaving storage to finishing transfusion
Red cells/whole blood	2–6°C	35 days	5 hours
Platelets	20–24°C on agitator rack	5 days	Consult supplier
Fresh frozen plasma	–30°C	1 year frozen	4 hours after thawing
Cryoprecipitate	–30°C	1 year frozen	4 hours after thawing

Blood filters

All blood products should be given through an appropriate giving set with an integral filter. Whole blood, packed cells, fresh frozen plasma and cryoprecipitate can be given through a blood giving set while platelets require a special giving set.

Blood warmers

If cold blood is infused too quickly, cardiac arrest can occur. Blood warmers should have a visible thermometer and audible alarm. If red cells and plasma are exposed to temperatures in excess of 40°C, severe transfusion reactions can occur. Blood should not be warmed by any other method.

Transfusion

During the transfusion of the blood product, observe the patient for signs of incompatibility or adverse reaction, e.g. fever, flushing, vomiting, urticaria, diarrhoea, itching, headache, rigors, haemoglobinuria, severe backache, pain at transfusion site, collapse, circulatory failure. If any of these signs are observed, stop the transfusion, inform the doctor and keep the intravenous line open with normal saline. Acute haemolytic transfusion reactions can be fatal and the patient may require epinephrine and chlorpheniramine.

Special requirements – premature babies

In pre-term babies a formal cross-match may be considered unnecessary in the first 4 months of life if there are no passively acquired maternal antibodies. CMV-negative, blood group O, Rhesus-negative blood with low anti-A and anti-B titres is usually provided in neonatal units and is suitable for neonates of any ABO and Rhesus D group.

Red cells must be transfused through a 20 μm filter to remove microaggregates.

PLATELET DISORDERS

Thrombocytopenia is caused by a reduction in platelet production or excessive peripheral destruction. Common causes of thrombocytopenia found in children are listed in Box 8.1.

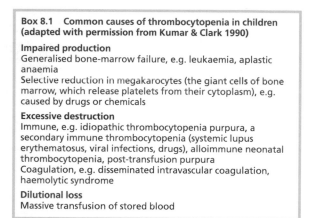

Box 8.1   Common causes of thrombocytopenia in children (adapted with permission from Kumar & Clark 1990)

Impaired production
Generalised bone-marrow failure, e.g. leukaemia, aplastic anaemia
Selective reduction in megakarocytes (the giant cells of bone marrow, which release platelets from their cytoplasm), e.g. caused by drugs or chemicals

Excessive destruction
Immune, e.g. idiopathic thrombocytopenia purpura, a secondary immune thrombocytopenia (systemic lupus erythematosus, viral infections, drugs), alloimmune neonatal thrombocytopenia, post-transfusion purpura
Coagulation, e.g. disseminated intravascular coagulation, haemolytic syndrome

Dilutional loss
Massive transfusion of stored blood

Disseminated intravascular coagulation is discussed as this may be seen in children presenting to paediatric intensive care or may develop, e.g. secondary to meningococcal disease.

Disseminated intravascular coagulation (DIC)

Disseminated intravascular coagulation refers to a spectrum of haemostatic disorders characterised by a reduction in factor V, factor VIII, fibrinogen and platelets. Wide-

---

Box 8.2 Common causes of disseminated intravascular coagulation

- Sepsis
- Haemolytic transfusion reactions
- Burns
- Fresh water drowning
- Snake bites

---

spread intravascular coagulation occurs, with secondary activation of fibrinolysis caused by excessive production of thrombin.

Clinical presentation
A patient with DIC may have no obvious signs of bleeding, merely abnormal clotting results or may present acutely ill, in shock, tachycardic, hypotensive, bleeding from venepuncture sites, nose, mouth as well as having signs of pulmonary and cerebral bleeds. Tissue necrosis may occur as a result of thrombus in peripheral veins.

Patients with DIC have:

- decreased platelets
- low fibrinogen
- increased fibrin degradation product
- extended prothrombin time
- extended partial thromboplastin time
- abnormal factors V and VIII.

Treatment

- Treat primary disease or precipitant
- Give blood products as indicated.

The role of heparin is controversial and may be indicated in a predominantly thrombotic DIC. The indications for its use depend on individual unit policy.

SEVERE ELECTROLYTE IMBALANCE

Children may be admitted with or develop severe electrolyte imbalance in paediatric intensive care, which can have dangerous consequences and will need prompt and appropriate treatment. Three important electrolytes to consider are sodium, potassium and magnesium, and common causes of imbalance and resulting effects are listed in Table 8.7, with principles for treatment.

Table 8.7 Common causes, diagnosis and principles of treatment for severe electrolyte imbalance of sodium, potassium and magnesium (adapted with permission from Hinds & Watson 1996)

Electrolyte imbalance	Common causes	Diagnosis and principles of treatment
Hyponatraemia Plasma sodium <135 mmol/L	Water intoxication Depletion of total body sodium Diuretic therapy Renal disease End-stage liver disease Fluid loss from alimentary tract Water depletion Salt retention in acute renal failure Administration of excessive sodium ions	Severe water intoxication can lead to confusion, convulsions and coma (often when sodium <120 mmol/L) Intravascular volume may be depleted **Treatment:** ● Aim to increase plasma sodium by a maximum of 2 mmol/h Cerebral oedema can occur and plasma sodium should be reduced by no more than 2 mmol/h **Treatment:** ● Give hypotonic intravenous fluids ● Haemodialysis
Hypernatraemia Plasma sodium >145 mmol/L		
Hypokalaemia Plasma potassium <3.5 mmol/L	Inadequate replacement of excessive urinary or gastrointestinal losses Steroid or diuretic therapy (causes increased urinary potassium loss)	May notice ECG changes, i.e. ST segment depression, decreased T-wave amplitude Can cause supraventricular tachycardia, especially in presence of digoxin **Treatment:** ● Slow intravenous potassium infusion (maximum peripheral concentration 40 mmol/L, maximum infusion rate 0.5 mmol/kg/h*)
Hyperkalaemia Plasma potassium >5 mmol/L	Excessive potassium infusion Acute renal failure Massive blood transfusion	May notice ECG changes, i.e. peaked T-waves, widening QRS complexes, which can lead to bradycardia and asystole

Administration of suxamethonium to patients with tissue damage, e.g. burns, which releases potassium into the circulation

Treatment:
- Intravenous dextrose and insulin drives potassium into cells
- Alkalinisation with sodium bicarbonate and hyperventilation both help shift potassium into the intracellular compartment and enhance potassium excretion via the kidneys
- Slow intravenous administration of salbutamol promotes cellular uptake of potassium by cAMP activation of the sodium/potassium pump
- Slow intravenous injection of calcium chloride in an emergency situation will temporarily antagonise cardiac effects of hyperkalaemia
- Haemofiltration or haemodialysis

Hypomagnesaemia Plasma magnesium <0.65 mmol/L	Excessive use of diuretics Administration of insulin in diabetic ketoacidosis Large gastrointestinal losses Malabsorption Long term parenteral nutrition with insufficient magnesium supplement	Tetany, muscle wasting, cardiac arrhythmias **Treatment:** - Oral or intravenous magnesium supplement – dilute intravenous magnesium sulphate to a concentration of 10%, i.e. 100 mg in 1 mL (maximum concentration is 20% or 200 mg in 1 mL), and give at a rate not exceeding 10 mg/kg/min*
Hypermagnesaemia Plasma magnesium >0.95 mmol/L	Excessive magnesium administration Renal failure	ECG changes, i.e. prolonged PR interval and QRS complexes, peaked T waves Hyporeflexia, respiratory paralysis, coma and cardiac arrest **Treatment:** - Intravenous administration of calcium chloride as an emergency to treat cardiac conduction defects – haemofiltration or haemodialysis

* *Guy's, St Thomas' and Lewisham Hospitals 1999*
cAMP: cyclic adenosine monophosphate.

REFERENCES

Dacie J V, Lewis S M 1997 Practical haematology, 8th edn. Churchill Livingstone, Edinburgh

Halliday H L, McClure G, Reid M 1985 Handbook of neonatal intensive care, 2nd edn. Baillière Tindall, Eastbourne

Hinds C J, Watson D 1996 Intensive care: a concise textbook, 2nd edn. W B Saunders, London

Kumar P J, Clark M L 1990 Clinical medicine, 2nd edn. Baillière Tindall, London

McClelland B (ed) 1996 Handbook of transfusion medicine. Blood Transfusion Services of the United Kingdom, 2nd edn. HMSO, London

Shann F 1996 Drug doses, 9th edn. Collective Pty Ltd, Australia

FURTHER READING

Blumer J L 1990 Pediatric intensive care, 3rd edn. C V Mosby, St Louis, MO

DRUGS – INOTROPES AND INFUSIONS

9

This chapter is intended for use as a quick reference guide and is not designed to replace the British National Formulary, the Association of the British Pharmaceutical Industry Data Sheet Compendium, paediatric formularies or any other sources of specialist information about drug use in children.

Great care has been taken to ensure that the dosages given are correct at the time of writing but dose schedules do change and relevant information sources should be used to check doses when necessary.

RESUSCITATION DRUGS

Drugs that may be used during resuscitation are outlined in Table 9.1.

Guidance regarding the indications for each of these drugs should be sought before use.

Table 9.1 Resuscitation drugs		
Drug	**Use**	**Intravenous dose**
Atropine sulphate	Sinus bradycardia	20 µg/kg*
Calcium chloride 10%	Acute hypotension	0.1–0.2 mL/kg
Epinephrine (adrenaline)	Cardiac arrest: initial dose	0.1 mL/kg of 1:10 000†
	subsequent doses	0.1 mL/kg of 1:1000‡
Lidocaine (lignocaine) 1%	Ventricular tachycardia	0.5–1 mg/kg
Sodium bicarbonate 8.4%	Correction of metabolic acidosis	1 mL/kg
Naloxone	Reversal of opioid induced respiratory depression	10 µg/kg

*The **minimum** dose of atropine sulphate that should be given is 100 µg to produce vagolytic effects and avoid paradoxical bradycardia (American Heart Association 1997)*
† Epinephrine 1:10 000 is equivalent to epinephrine 1 mg in 10 mL
‡ Epinephrine 1:1000 is equivalent to epinephrine 1 mg in 1 mL

See Chapter 1 for details of drugs that can be given via the endotracheal route.

DRUGS FOR INTUBATION

To reduce the risk of damaging the upper airway during intubation, infants and children should be sedated and paralysed prior to the procedure. The sedatives and neuromuscular blocking drugs commonly used as premedication for intubation are outlined in Table 9.2. Comprehensive prescribing information should be consulted before prescribing or administering these drugs.

Table 9.2 Drugs for intubation (drug doses from Guy's, St Thomas' and Lewisham Hospitals 1999)

Drug	Intravenous dose	Notes and rationale
Atracurium – a non-depolarising neuromuscular blocking agent	Initially 300–600 µg/kg	Often drug of choice in patients with renal or hepatic impairment Can cause histamine release so avoid in asthma Short to intermediate duration of action
Ketamine – a general anaesthetic agent	1–2 mg/kg	Contraindicated in hypertension Incidence of hallucinations is higher in older children and teenagers Coadministration of a benzodiazepine reduces the incidence of hallucinations
Midazolam – a benzodiazepine used for sedation	100–200 µg/kg	Can cause respiratory depression with severe hypotension (this effect is potentiated by coadministration of erythromycin)
Morphine – an opioid sedative and analgesic	50–100 µg/kg 100–200 µg/kg	In neonates Over 1 month Neonates and infants show increased susceptibility to respiratory depression
Pancuronium – a non-polarising neuromuscular blocking agent	30–40 µg/kg 60–100 µg/kg	In neonates In children Long duration of action (60–120 min) No histamine release but can cause tachycardia and hypertension

		Use with caution in severe renal and liver failure as duration is prolonged
Suxamethonium – a depolarising neuromuscular blocking agent	2 mg/kg 1–2 mg/kg Maximum total dose 100 mg	In neonates and infants In children Very rapid onset of action (60 s) Short duration of action (4–6 min) May cause bradycardia in children, especially following a second dose Not recommended in liver disease, burns or in patients with Duchenne muscular dystrophy Can cause profound hyperkalaemia, especially in burns, trauma and in patients with renal failure
Thiopentone – used for induction of anaesthesia	2–7 mg/kg	Acutely reduces intracranial pressure and reduces cerebral metabolism, so may be drug of choice in patients with a head injury (Singer & Webb 1997)

QUICK REFERENCE GUIDE FOR CALCULATING INFUSIONS

Many units use standard infusion calculations. Table 9.3 shows some of these 'rules of thumb' for frequently used drugs in paediatric intensive care.

These are not designed to replace infusion checking calculations which must always be performed when making up infusions. All infusions are made up to 50 mL.

Checking the infusion dose from the syringe concentration:

- Use the prescribed drug dose, i.e. the total amount in the 50 mL syringe × 1000 to give amount in nanograms or micrograms
- Divide this by 50 to give the amount per millilitre
- Divide by the weight in kilograms to give amount per kilogram per millilitre
- (Divide this figure by 60 if the infusion is calculated dose/kg/min).

Table 9.3	Standard preparation for intravenous drug infusions		
Drug	**Quantity in 50 mL syringe**	**Diluent**	**Dose if infusion run at 1 mL/h**
Aminophylline	50 mg × weight (kg)	0.9% saline or 5% dextrose to 50 mL	1 mg/kg/h
Dinoprostone (prostaglandin E₂)	30 **micrograms** × weight (kg)	0.9% saline or 5% dextrose to 50 mL	10 **nanograms**/kg/min
Dobutamine	30 mg × weight (kg)	0.9% saline or 5% dextrose to 50 mL	10 µg/kg/min
Dopamine	30 mg × weight (kg)	0.9% saline or 5% dextrose to 50 mL	10 µg/kg/min
Epinephrine (adrenaline)	3 mg × weight (kg)	0.9% saline or 5% dextrose to 50 mL	1 µg/kg/min
Frusemide	25 mg × weight (kg)	0.9% saline to 50 mL	0.5 mg/kg/h
Glyceryl trinitrate	3 mg × weight (kg)	0.9% saline or 5% dextrose to 50 mL	1 µg/kg/min
Midazolam	3 mg × weight (kg)	0.9% saline or 5% dextrose to 50 mL	1 µg/kg/min
Morphine	1 mg × weight (kg)	0.9% saline or 5% dextrose to 50 mL	20 µg/kg/h
Norepinephrine (noradrenaline)	3 mg × weight (kg)	0.9% saline or 5% dextrose to 50 mL	1 µg/kg/min
Salbutamol	3 mg × weight (kg)	0.9% saline or 5% dextrose to 50 mL	1 µg/kg/min
Sodium nitroprusside*	3 mg × weight (kg)	0.9% saline or 5% dextrose to 50 mL	1 µg/kg/min
Vecuronium	5 mg × weight (kg)	0.9% saline or 5% dextrose to 50 mL	100 µg/kg/h

* Sodium nitroprusside when made up must be protected from light and if available an amber giving set can be used

Take great care to ensure that the correct units are used in the calculation.

INOTROPIC AND CHRONOTROPIC DRUGS

An inotrope is a drug that alters the force of cardiac muscular contraction.

Table 9.4 The pharmacological effect and receptor selectivity of various inotropic and chronotropic drugs (reproduced with permission from Young & Koda-Kimble 1995)

	Receptor selectivity			Pharmacological effect		Inotropic	Chronotropic
	α	β₁	β₂	Peripheral vascular vasodilation	Peripheral vascular vasoconstriction		
Dobutamine	+	+++	++	++	-	++	+
Dopamine 0.5–2 µg/kg/min	-	-	-	- (renal and splanchnic dilatation)	-	-	-
Dopamine 2–5 µg/kg/min	-	+	-	- (renal and splanchnic dilatation)	+	+	+
Dopamine > 5 µg/kg/min	+	++	-	- (renal and splanchnic dilatation)	++	++	++
Enoximone	-	-	-	+	-	+++	+
Epinephrine	+	+++	++	++	-	+++	++
Isoprenaline	-	+++	+++	+++	-	++	++
Norepinephrine	++++	++	-	-	++++	+	+

A chronotrope is a drug that alters the heart rate, i.e. the rate of contraction of the heart.

Inotropic and chronotropic drugs are used in clinical practice. The effects produced by inotropic and chronotropic drugs are largely dependent upon the receptor sites activated and the doses administered. Table 9.4 outlines the receptor selectivity and pharmacological effects produced by commonly used agents.

DRUGS COMMONLY USED AS INTRAVENOUS INFUSIONS (URQUHART 1998, PERSONAL COMMUNICATION)

Drugs included: aminophylline, amiodarone, dinoprostone, dobutamine, dopamine, enoximone, epinephrine (adrenaline), frusemide, glyceryl trinitrate, midazolam, morphine, norepinephrine (noradrenaline), salbutamol, sodium nitroprusside, vecuronium.

Adrenaline

See epinephrine.

Aminophylline

Pharmacology: Aminophylline is a combination of theophylline and ethylenediamine. This combination has the advantage of increased solubility compared to theophylline. Theophylline is an inhibitor of cyclic adenosine mono-phosphate (cAMP) phosphodiesterase and is an adenosine receptor antagonist. The most clinically useful pharmacological effect is its potent bronchodilator activity.

Indications: Reversible airways disease, severe acute asthma.

Monitoring: Monitoring of plasma concentrations is necessary as theophylline's pharmacokinetics show large interpatient variation, its metabolism can be altered by other drugs and chemicals, and the blood levels likely to cause toxicity are close to those required to produce beneficial effects.

Side effects: Hypokalaemia (particularly in combination with β_2-receptor agonists), tachycardia, palpitations, gastrointestinal disturbances, arrhythmias and, in overdose, convulsions.

Intravenous infusion

- Infuse centrally or peripherally
- May be diluted with 0.9% saline or 5% dextrose

- $50\,mg \times$ body weight (kg) in $50\,mL \rightarrow 1\,mL/hour$
  $= 1\,mg/kg/h$.

Amiodarone

Pharmacology: Amiodarone is a class III anti-arrhythmic drug that is useful in the treatment of supraventricular tachycardia and ventricular arrhythmias. Its main mechanism of action is prolongation of the refractory period. It has the advantage of causing little or no myocardial depression. It acts rapidly when given by intravenous infusion and has a very long elimination half-life, particularly after chronic treatment.

Indications: Treatment of arrhythmias, particularly when other drugs are contraindicated or ineffective.

Monitoring: Liver and thyroid function tests should be performed on prolonged oral therapy and during intravenous therapy. Electrocardiograph and blood pressure monitoring are mandatory. Monitoring of plasma concentrations can be useful.

Side effects: Intravenous amiodarone can produce a drop in blood pressure, particularly if infused too rapidly. Hepatotoxicity, thyroid disturbances, peripheral neuropathy, pulmonary toxicity, corneal microdeposits and phototoxicity may all occur during chronic therapy.

Intravenous infusion
- Infuse centrally if possible, as peripheral infusions are likely to cause thrombophlebitis
- May be diluted with 5% dextrose – do not use 0.9% saline
- When diluted, amiodarone should be diluted to at least $600\,\mu g/mL$.

Dinoprostone (prostaglandin E₂)

Pharmacology: Dinoprostone is derived from the unsaturated long-chain fatty acid arachidonic acid, by the cyclo-oxygenase enzyme system, the enzyme inhibited by non-steroidal anti-inflammatory drugs. Dinoprostone has a variety of pharmacological actions, including vascular smooth muscle relaxation, stimulation of uterine contractions, alteration in renal blood flow resulting in diuresis and involvement in inflammatory responses.

Indications: Dinoprostone is most commonly used in paediatrics to maintain the patency of the ductus arteriosus in neonates with congenital heart defects until corrective surgery is possible. Alprostadil (prostaglandin E₁) can also be used for this purpose. Alprostadil is licensed for this indication but is, however, considerably more expensive.

Monitoring: Arterial blood pressure, oxygen saturation; facilities for intubation and ventilation should be available.

Side effects: Intravenous dinoprostone can cause apnoea and respiratory depression. Other side effects include hypotension, flushing, bradycardia, tachycardia and oedema.

Intravenous infusion
- Infuse centrally or peripherally; if a peripheral line is used, ensure that other intravenous access is available if the line tissues
- May be diluted with 0.9% saline or 5% dextrose
- $30\,\mu g \times$ body weight (kg) in $50\,mL \rightarrow 1\,mL/h =$ 10 nanograms /kg/min.

Dobutamine

Pharmacology: Dobutamine is made up of two stereoisomers: D-dobutamine and L-dobutamine. These isomers have different pharmacological activity and their combined activity is responsible for the effects produced by dobutamine. D-dobutamine stimulates β_1-adrenoreceptors to increase cardiac contractility and β_2-adrenoreceptors to cause vasodilation in mesenteric and skeletal vascular beds. L-dobutamine stimulates α_1-adrenoreceptors to cause vasoconstriction. The vasodilatory and vasoconstricting effects counterbalance each other and the primary haemodynamic response during dobutamine infusion is an increase in cardiac output, with little change in blood pressure. Dobutamine has no effect upon dopamine receptors.

Indications: Inotropic support in cardiac surgery, cardiomyopathy, septic shock and cardiogenic shock.

Monitoring: Arterial blood pressure, heart rate and continuous ECG.

Side effects: Tachycardia, hypotension, systolic hypertension, arrhythmia, extravasation injury.

Intravenous infusion
- Infuse via central line whenever possible
- May be diluted with 0.9% saline or 5% dextrose
- 30 mg × body weight (kg) in 50 mL → 1 mL/h = $10\,\mu g/kg/min$.

Dopamine

Pharmacology: The cardiovascular effects of dopamine are mediated by its stimulation of a number of different receptor types: dopamine D_1 and D_2 receptors; β_1-adrenoreceptors; and α_1-adrenoreceptors.

At low doses ($0.5–2\,\mu g/kg/min$) the predominant action of dopamine is to stimulate vascular dopamine D_1 receptors, causing vasodilation in mesenteric, renal and coronary vascular beds. The resulting increase in renal blood flow and glomerular filtration rate is the basis of the so called 'renal' dopamine effect. At medium doses ($2–5\,\mu g/kg/min$) the effects produced by stimulation of β_1-adrenoreceptors are added. Thus, positive inotropic and chronotropic effects usually result in increased systolic blood pressure and pulse pressure with no effect or a small increase in diastolic pressure.

At higher doses ($>5\,\mu g/kg/minute$) dopamine activates α_1-adrenoreceptors, causing vasoconstriction. Thus, increases in systemic vascular resistance, systolic and diastolic blood pressure and a reduced renal dopamine effect are seen.

Indications: Inotropic therapy in cardiogenic shock.

Monitoring: Arterial blood pressure, heart rate and continuous ECG.

Side effects: Peripheral vasoconstriction, hypertension, tachycardia, extravasation injury.

Intravenous infusion
- Infuse via central line whenever possible
- Peripheral infusion of dopamine causes vasoconstriction; high doses may result in gangrene and significant extravasation injury
- May be diluted with 0.9% saline or 5% dextrose
- 30 mg × body weight (kg) in 50 mL → 1 mL/h = $10\,\mu g/kg/min$.

Enoximone

Pharmacology: Enoximone is a selective inhibitor of phosphodiesterase III (PDEIII). This is the enzyme that is responsible for catalysing the breakdown of cyclic adenosine monophosphate (cAMP). Inhibition of PDEIII results in accumulation of cAMP. PDEIII is found in high concentrations in cardiac and vascular smooth muscle. Administration of enoximone results in high cAMP levels in cardiac and vascular smooth muscle. This causes positive inotropy and vasodilation. Enoximone is therefore a positive inotrope-vasodilator.

Indications: Congestive cardiac failure where cardiac output is reduced and filling pressures are increased.

Monitoring: Arterial blood pressure, heart rate and continuous ECG.

Side effects: Arrhythmias, hypotension

Intravenous infusion
- Infuse centrally or peripherally
- Unstable in solution, only dilute with an equal volume of water for injection or 0.9% saline; do not dilute with any other diluents or use any other concentrations
- Avoid mixing with other infusions
- Injection may be given orally.

Epinephrine (adrenaline)

Pharmacology: Epinephrine is a potent stimulator of α-, β_1- and β_2-adrenoreceptors and has low affinity for dopamine receptors. The effects it produces are dependent upon this receptor sensitivity. β_1-receptor stimulation produces positive inotropy, increasing systolic blood pressure and cardiac output. β_2-receptor stimulation produces skeletal muscle vasodilation, which results in reduced peripheral vascular resistance and often a fall in diastolic blood pressure. At higher doses, α_1-receptor stimulation becomes increasingly significant and produces peripheral vasoconstriction, resulting in increases in peripheral resistance and diastolic blood pressure.

Indications: Inotropic therapy in cardiogenic shock.

Monitoring: Arterial blood pressure, heart rate and continuous ECG.

Side effects: Tachycardia, arrhythmias, hypertension, extravasation injury.

Intravenous infusion
- When used as an infusion, epinephrine should be infused via a central line wherever possible because of the risk of vasoconstriction and extravasation injury
- May be diluted with 0.9% saline or 5% dextrose
- $3\,mg \times$ body weight (kg) in $50\,mL \to 1\,mL/h = 1\,\mu g/kg/min$.

Frusemide

Pharmacology: Frusemide is a loop diuretic that inhibits electrolyte reabsorption from the ascending limb of the loop of Henle in the renal tubules. It can be useful in renal failure when other groups of diuretics are ineffective but can cause electrolyte disturbances, particularly hypokalaemia.

Indications: Oedema, oliguria due to renal failure.

Monitoring: Fluid balance, blood urea and electrolytes and blood pressure.

Side effects: Hyponatraemia, hypokalaemia, hypomagnesaemia, increased calcium excretion, hypotension, tinnitus and deafness (particularly in renal failure, large parenteral doses and rapid administration).

Intravenous infusion
- Infuse peripherally or centrally
- May be diluted with 0.9% saline
- The neat injection has a concentration of 10 mg/mL
- $25\,mg \times$ body weight (kg) in $50\,mL \to 1\,mL/h = 0.5\,mg/kg/h$.

Glyceryl trinitrate

Pharmacology: Glyceryl trinitrate produces smooth muscle relaxation and as a result it is a powerful vasodilator of both arterial and venous vasculature. Its effects are mediated by nitric oxide released when glyceryl trinitrate is metabolised. It is a powerful antihypertensive agent and reduces afterload in cardiac failure. Tolerance to the effects of glyceryl trinitrate often develops after continuous prolonged use.

Indications: Left ventricular failure.

Monitoring: Blood pressure, heart rate, methaemoglobin concentrations.

Side effects: Headache, hypotension, tachycardia, methaemoglobinaemia.

Intravenous infusion
- Infuse peripherally or centrally
- May be diluted with 0.9% saline or 5% dextrose
- The neat solution has a concentration of 1 mg/mL
- 3 mg × body weight (kg) in 50 mL → 1 mL/h = 1 μg/kg/min.

Midazolam

Pharmacology: Midazolam is a short-acting benzodiazepine that binds to benzodiazepine receptors in the central nervous system to produce a variety of effects, including sedation, anxiolysis, anticonvulsant effects and amnesia. Effects may be reversed by the benzodiazepine antagonist flumazenil, although this is rarely necessary.

Indications: Sedation, premedication, treatment of epilepsy.

Monitoring: Arterial blood pressure, oxygen saturation.

Side effects: Respiratory depression and severe hypotension after intravenous administration, acute withdrawal syndrome after prolonged use (1–2 weeks).

Intravenous infusion
- Infuse peripherally or centrally
- May be diluted with 0.9% saline or 5% dextrose
- The neat injection has a maximum concentration of 5 mg/mL
- 3 mg × body weight (kg) in 50 mL → 1 mL/h = 1 μg/kg/minute.

Morphine

Pharmacology: Morphine is an agonist of a number of morphine receptor subtypes. Its most important therapeutic and adverse effects are thought to be mediated via μ- and κ-opioid receptors. Morphine produces a wide range of pharmacological effects, including analgesia, sedation, respiratory depression, euphoria, inhibition of gut motility, miosis, nausea and vomiting.

Indications: Analgesia, sedation.

Monitoring: Sedation, respiratory rate, oxygen saturation.

Side effects: Nausea and vomiting, constipation, respiratory depression (especially neonates), hypotension, miosis, hallucinations, acute withdrawal syndrome after prolonged use.

Intravenous infusion
- Infuse peripherally or centrally
- May be diluted with 0.9% saline or 5% dextrose
- 1 mg × body weight (kg) in 50 mL → 1 mL/h = 20 µg/kg/h.

Norepinephrine (noradrenaline)

Pharmacology: Norepinephrine is a potent stimulator of α-adrenoreceptors and when given intravenously the effects produced are predominantly α-mediated. Infusions produce vasoconstriction with an increase in systemic vascular resistance and an elevation of both systolic and diastolic blood pressure. Cardiac output is usually unchanged or reduced. Blood flow to most vascular beds is reduced, including the kidney and the liver.

Indications: Acute hypotension.

Monitoring: Arterial blood pressure, heart rate and continuous ECG.

Side effects: Hypertension, arrhythmias, peripheral ischaemia, extravasation injury.

Intravenous infusion
- Infuse via a central line as norepinephrine is a very potent vasoconstrictor
- Extravasation may cause tissue necrosis
- May be diluted with 0.9% saline or 5% dextrose
- Doses should be calculated in terms of norepinephrine base
- 3 mg × body weight (kg) in 50 mL → 1 mL/h – 1 µg/kg/min.

Prostaglandin E$_2$

See Dinoprostone.

Salbutamol

Pharmacology: Salbutamol is a selective β$_2$-adrenoceptor agonist. It is useful principally as a bronchodilator, although other effects such as reducing serum potassium are clinically beneficial.

Indications: Reversible airways disease, renal hyperkalaemia.

Monitoring: ECG, serum potassium, heart rate, oxygen saturation.

Side effects: Peripheral vasodilation, tachycardia, hypo-kalaemia.

Intravenous infusion
- Infuse peripherally or centrally
- May be diluted with 0.9% saline or 5% dextrose
- 3 mg × body weight (kg) in 50 mL → 1 mL/h = 1 μg/kg/min.

Sodium nitroprusside (Nipride)

Pharmacology: Sodium nitroprusside produces smooth muscle relaxation and as a result it is a powerful vasodilator of both arterial and venous vasculature. It is effective as an antihypertensive and to reduce preload in cardiac failure. Its effects are mediated by nitric oxide, produced as a result of the spontaneous breakdown of nitroprusside. Tolerance is less likely to develop after prolonged use of nitroprusside than with other nitrates. Breakdown of nitroprusside results in the production of thiocyanate, which may accumulate after prolonged infusion.

Indications: Hypertensive crisis, left ventricular failure.

Monitoring: Blood pressure, heart rate, methaemoglobin concentrations, serum thiocyanate levels (after 72 h of infusion).

Side effects: Hypotension, headache, tachycardia, symptoms of rapid blood pressure reduction.

Intravenous infusion
- Infuse peripherally or centrally
- Must be reconstituted with 5% dextrose. It is usually further diluted to 200 μg/mL with 0.9% saline or 5% dextrose.

Vecuronium

Pharmacology: Vecuronium bromide is a non-depolarising neuromuscular blocking agent with a high degree of selectivity for the nicotinic acetylcholine receptors. Its effects may be reversed by the use of an anticholinesterase drug such as neostigmine. Following an intravenous bolus dose, it has an onset of action of about 2 min and lasts for 15–20 min in children and 30–40 min in infants. It

Table 9.5 Therapeutic drug monitoring (reproduced with permission from R Urquhart, personal communication, 1998)

Drug	Recommended sample time	Target range	Time to steady state (approx.)	Sample bottle	Notes
Aminophylline	Infusion: 6–12 h after starting then every 24 h	10–20 mg/L (theophylline)	24–48 h	Plain (clotted)	Assay is for theophylline
Carbamazepine	Before dose	4–14 mg/L	2–4 weeks after starting, then 3–4 d after each dose change	Plain (clotted)	
Digoxin	> 6 h post-dose	0.8–2.2 µg/L	5–10 d	Plain (clotted)	
Gentamicin 'once daily'	18 h post-dose	< 1 mg/L	24 h	Plain (clotted)	Resample after 6–12 h if > 1 mg/L
Gentamicin 'conventional'	Peak: 60 min post-dose Trough: before dose	Peak: 6–10 mg/L Trough: < 2 mg/L	24 h	Plain (clotted)	
Phenobarbitone	Before dose	9–40 mg/L	14 d	Plain (clotted)	
Phenytoin	IV: > 60 min post-dose PO: before dose	10–20 mg/L	1–2 weeks (very variable)	Plain (clotted)	Seek advice if albumin binding is altered
Vancomycin	Trough: before dose	Trough: 5–10 mg/L	24–36 h	Plain (clotted)	

rarely causes histamine release and has good cardiovascular stability.

Indications: Neuromuscular blockade.

Monitoring: Peripheral nerve stimulator; ventilation is mandatory.

Side effects: Recovery time is increased after prolonged use; very rare hypersensitivity reactions.

Intravenous infusion

- Infuse peripherally or centrally
- May be diluted with 0.9% saline or 5% dextrose
- Upon standard reconstitution the injection concentration is 2 mg/mL. However, vecuronium may be infused at concentrations up to 4 mg/mL. If necessary, reconstitute using half the recommended volume to produce the 4 mg/mL solution.
- 5 mg × body weight (kg) in 50 mL → 1 mL/h = 100 μg/kg/h.

THERAPEUTIC DRUG MONITORING

Measurement of plasma levels is necessary for a range of drugs with a narrow therapeutic index. These drugs have a minimum therapeutic concentration that is close to their minimum toxic concentration. The target ranges of concentrations for these drugs are displayed in Table 9.5 (p. 157). The receptor selectivity and pharmacological effects produced by commonly used agents are shown in Table 9.4 (p. 157). It may be necessary at times to run intravenous infusions concurrently and, while this should only be practised where absolutely essential, Table 9.6 shows intravenous compatabilities known.

Table 9.6 Intravenous compatibilities (reproduced with permission from Guy's, St Thomas' and Lewisham Hospitals 1999)

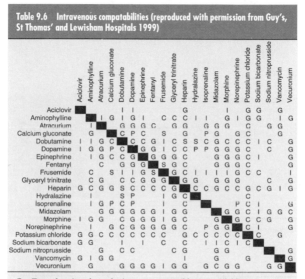

	Aciclovir	Aminophylline	Atracurium	Calcium gluconate	Dobutamine	Dopamine	Epinephrine	Fentanyl	Frusemide	Glyceryl trinitrate	Heparin	Hydralazine	Isoprenaline	Midazolam	Morphine	Norepinephrine	Potassium chloride	Sodium bicarbonate	Sodium nitroprusside	Vancomycin	Vecuronium
Aciclovir	■				I	I					G			I			G	G		G	
Aminophylline		■	I	G	I	G	I			C	C	C			I		G	I	G	G		G
Atracurium		I	■		G	G	G	C		G	G		G	G	G		C			G	G	G
Calcium gluconate	G			■	C	P	C		S		G		P	G		G	C			G	
Dobutamine	I	I	G	C	■		C	C	G	I	C	S	S	C	G	C	C	C	I		C	G
Dopamine	I	G	G	P	C	■	G	G	I		C	C	P	P	G	G	G	C		C		G
Epinephrine		I		G	C	C	■	G	G	C			G	G	G	C		I			G
Fentanyl		C			G	G	G	■	S	G	C			G	G	G	C				G
Frusemide	C		S		I	I	G	S	■	G	C		I	I	I	G	C	C		I	
Glyceryl trinitrate	C	G		C	C	G	G	G	G	■	G	G		G	G	G			C		G
Heparin	G	C	G	G	S	C	C	C	C	G	■	C	C	G	C	C	G	C	G	I	G
Hydralazine		I			S	P				I	G	C						C			
Isoprenaline		I		G	P	C	P			I			C			P	C	I			G
Midazolam	I		G	G	G	G	G	G	I		G	G		■		G	G	C	I	G	G	C
Morphine	I	G	G		C	G	G	G	I		G	C		G	■	G	C	C	G		G
Norepinephrine		I		G	C	G	G	G	G	C		P	G	G		■	C	I			G
Potassium chloride	G	G	C	C	C	C	C	C	C		G	C	C	C	C	C	■	C		G	
Sodium bicarbonate	G	G			I				C			I	I	C	I		C	■			
Sodium nitroprusside			G		C	C				C	G			G	G				■		G
Vancomycin	G	I	G	G							I						G			■	G
Vecuronium		G			G	G	G	I		G	G			G	C	G	G		G	G	■

C = Data showing that solutions are compatible are available.
P = Although the manufacturers do not provide information on compatabilities these solutions have been used in practice without problems; check for precipitation or colour change during use.
S = Compatible in sodium chloride 0.9% only. G = Compatible in glucose solutions only. I = Incompatible.

REFERENCES

American Heart Association 1997 Pediatric advanced life support. American Heart Association , Dallas, TX: p 6–9

Guy's, St Thomas' and Lewisham Hospitals 1999 Paediatric formulary, 5th edn. Guy's, St Thomas' and Lewisham Hospitals, London

Singer M, Webb A 1997 Oxford handbook of critical care. Oxford University Press, Oxford: p 232

Young L Y, Koda-Kimble M A (eds) 1995 Applied therapeutics, 6th edn. Applied Therapeutics, Vancouver, BC: p 18–12

While it is acknowledged that all management will be according to local policies, these guidelines may be helpful.

CROUP (LARYNGOTRACHEOBRONCHITIS)

If intubation is required to maintain a secure airway:

- Wean ventilation and allow child to self-ventilate via a Swedish nose filter on the end of the ET tube
- Secureness of tube is vital – tapes may need to be changed daily because of secretions and movement of child
- Use of arm splints effective in preventing self extubation
- Regular suction – if child is active, likely to cough up secretions frequently
- Child is likely to be on a course of steroids from admission to PICU – wait to hear leak around tube prior to extubation, can take 3–5 days
- Importance of play, involvement of family in care and daily routine to minimise distress and boredom while ET tube is in situ.

STATUS ASTHMATICUS

- Ventilation is avoided if possible – difficulties caused by prolonged expiration phase. Give O_2, nebulised and IV bronchodilators (salbutamol/aminophylline) and steroids.

- If ventilated, attempt to keep child sedated (morphine/fentanyl infusions) but not paralysed and use a pressure/volume support mode in order to assist, rather than take over, the child's own breathing pattern. Consider permissive hypercapnia.

- If unable to ventilate effectively, use muscle relaxant drugs (avoiding those causing histamine release, e.g. atracurium) in conjunction with sedation and fully ventilate. Use a slow rate with prolonged expiration phase to facilitate expiration and limit air trapping. Second-line drugs with bronchodilator properties may be used: propofol/ketamine.

• Monitor potassium levels closely if salbutamol is used – potassium replacement may be necessary.

DIABETIC KETOACIDOSIS (DKA)

DKA is a state of hypertonic dehydration and metabolic decompensation that results from inadequate levels of insulin in the body.

• Problems include:
  – Hyperglycaemia
  – Ketoacidaemia
  – Acid–base disturbance
  – Electrolyte disturbances
• Leading causes of death in children with DKA:
  – Cerebral oedema
  – Hypokalaemia
  – Inhalation of vomit.

Airway – Breathing – Circulation

• Fluid management – RAPID treatment of hypovolaemia with SLOW correction of dehydration
• Reversal of abnormal metabolism with insulin – hourly blood sugar monitoring with continuous IV infusion of insulin titrated to blood sugar levels
• Careful monitoring and correction of electrolytes – particularly potassium; monitor ECG
• Bicarbonate may be necessary to correct acidosis
• Frequent clinical and laboratory monitoring to reassess condition and response to treatment
• Urinalysis – particularly ketones and glucose; urine mc & s
• Hourly neuro assessment (more frequently if indicated).

BURNS

• Four main categories:
  – Thermal
  – Chemical
  – Electrical
  – Radiation.

Airway – Breathing – Circulation

• *Inhalational injury* – Direct, causing damage to mucosa and underlying tissues – resulting oedema carries risk of airway obstruction. Indirect via smoke inhalation may cause inflammation and ulceration in upper airway, trachea and large bronchi, carries risk of pneumonia and ARDS developing

24–48 h post-injury. Carbon monoxide (CO) from smoke combines with haemoglobin to form carboxyhaemoglobin (COHb), incapable of transporting O_2 to the tissues; important to ascertain the level of COHb in the bloodstream. SaO_2 ineffective – co-oximeter reading will give accurate COHb level. Give 100% humidified O_2. High-frequency oscillation ventilation (HFOV) may be considered if the child is difficult to ventilate, to reduce the risk of barotrauma.

• *Assessment of burns* – Lund and Browder chart frequently used, or patient's palm equals 1% body surface area (BSA). Assess depth – superficial/partial/full-thickness. Escharotomy may be performed for compartment syndrome.

• *Fluid resuscitation* – various formulae, e.g. Parkland Formula advocated by Scilley (1997):
  – 4 mL/kg/%burn within first 24 h
  – Add this fluid to the daily maintenance fluid for 24 h
  – Half of the total amount of this fluid to be given in the first 8 h
  – Remainder over the next 16 h.

  Evaluation of fluid resuscitation is based largely on urine output (more than 1 mL/kg/h) as well as vital signs, acid–base balance and lactate. Fluid should be crystalloid (0.9% saline or Hartmann's). Inotropic support may be required in children with burns covering more than 30–40% BSA. Colloid may be given at 8–12 hours – permeability changes may start to reverse.

• *Clean wounds* (0.9% saline commonly used) – Variety of clean dressings promoting moist wound healing, e.g. paraffin gauze and bandages. Local policies differ. Elevate burnt hands in slings. Avoid heat loss. Culture regularly and treat infection with appropriate antibiotics. Facilitate wound closure.

• *Pain management*

• *Enteral feeds* should be introduced as soon as possible – monitor weight, calorie and protein intake. Various formulae used to calculate daily requirements (hypermetabolic state usually 3–5 days postinjury).

MULTIORGAN FAILURE

• Ventilation – lung protective strategies should be adopted:
  – HFOV may be required if conventional ventilation is insufficient.
  – Permissive hypercapnoea and hypoxaemia.
  – Prone positioning may improve lung perfusion and ventilation

- *Cardiac function* should be supported:
  - Correct preload with crystalloid/colloid
  - Inotropes – particularly dopamine and low dose norepinephrine/epinephrine (0.01–0.1 μg/kg/min)
- *Fluid management*:
  - Monitor CVP
  - Strict monitoring of fluid balance
  - May need to use CVVH to remove fluid
- *Renal function*:
  - Test urine (dipstick and mc&s)
  - Pay close attention to electrolytes and replace as necessary
  - As stated above, may need to use CVVH/CVVHD depending on urea/creatinine/potassium levels/degree of fluid overload/acid–base balance/pyrexia
- *Liver function*:
  - Child may have DIC – pay close attention to FBC and clotting results and administer blood/clotting products as necessary (Chapter 8)
  - Liver function tests (Chapter 5)
  - Monitor blood sugar levels
  - Monitor levels of routinely used drugs that are metabolised by the liver, e.g. morphine
- *Gastrointestinal function*:
  - Feed enterally if possible – if nasogastric feeds are not tolerated, many centres advocate continuing to deliver a very small amount of feed, e.g. 1 mL/h in an infant – extra to the fluid allowance – in order to promote gut motility
- *Neurological function*:
  - Hourly neuro assessment – easier to assess child if sedated but not paralysed
  - Risk of seizures – if child has to be paralysed consider use of CFAM
  - Consider risk of raised ICP, particularly if DIC is present
  - risk of cerebral bleed (Chapter 6)
- *Skin integrity*:
  - Critically ill child with poor peripheral perfusion is particularly at risk of skin breakdown – consider suitable mattresses/beds to promote effective pressure area care
- Give appropriate antibiotics and check that levels are within therapeutic range
- Care of the family is particularly important when managing these children – the prognosis may be poor

REFERENCE

Scilley CG 1997 Burn injury. In: Singh NC (ed) Manual of pediatric critical care. WB Saunders, Philadephia

PRINCIPLES OF SAFE TRANSPORT

In 1993 the report of a working party commissioned by the British Paediatric Association (BPA) recommended the reorganisation of paediatric intensive care units (PICUs) in the UK. At the present time, critically ill children may be looked after in a District General Hospital (DGH), adult intensive therapy or high-dependency unit, or transferred to a PICU. Measures designed to regionalise paediatric intensive care facilities are under way in many areas, following the recommendations made by the BPA (1993) and the Department of Health (DoH 1997a, b).

Although the vital role of the DGH in the stabilisation of critically ill children is widely acknowledged, an integral part of the above recommendations is the presence of dedicated intensivists and a paediatric retrieval team (PRT) to transfer patients safely to the tertiary unit. The value of the PRT in being able to deliver intensive care to seriously ill children even prior to transfer is emphasised (Britto et al 1995). By providing the monitoring facilities available in a PICU in a compact, mobile and reliable form in transit, the team should be able to ensure that there is no interruption to the patient's therapy, monitoring or medical and nursing care during a well planned and executed transport procedure (PICS 1996).

THE RETRIEVAL NURSE

It is acknowledged that the participation of nursing staff as members of the transfer team is essential; they act as skilled assistants to the medical staff and are able to assess the nursing needs of the child (PICS 1996). It is important that only experienced and appropriately trained nurses take on this role as a wide range of skills and expertise are required, in a difficult working environment without the assistance of colleagues. A confident, competent practitioner is required who can cope with the considerable demands of the role, and familiarity with the *Scope of Professional Practice* (UKCC 1992) is essential. It is recommended that only nurses with a higher qualification in paediatric intensive care – the ENB 415 or equivalent – should participate and that, in addition, in-house training should be provided for all those participating in retrievals (PICS 1996, DoH 1997b).

COMMUNICATION

One of the key skills required for a retrieval team to function smoothly and effectively is good communication; this is particularly important among the staff members of the PRT – usually one doctor and one nurse but possibly other staff/trainees accompanying them – enabling efficient teamwork to take place. This team then needs to communicate effectively with its base, the ambulance crew, the child and family and the staff at the referring hospital. Forming friendly, constructive relationships with the staff who have recognised the need to transfer the child to your unit and may have worked hard for many hours resuscitating and trying to stabilise a sick child is very important.

As well as training their own staff, it is envisaged that Lead Centres should develop into a resource providing advice and training covering their whole geographical area; by arranging placements for both doctors and nurses from centres that see relatively few critically ill children, opportunities for them to maintain their skills will be provided (DoH 1997a).

BEFORE YOU LEAVE

• All equipment should have been checked; monitors and pumps should be fully charged.

• Consider the age, size and provisional diagnosis of the child – do you need to take anything extra or, alternatively, could you leave anything behind? For example, if you are retrieving an infant, do you really need to take a range of large ET tubes just because they are part of the standard kit?

• Regardless of the contents of your kit, many people find it invaluable to have scissors, a few plain labels, pens, a calculator and a roll of clear tape in their pockets.

• The doctor will have discussed the child with staff at the referring unit and possibly given them advice on further management while they await the team's arrival. Check that the location of the child within the referring hospital is documented, together with directions if appropriate, as this can save valuable time.

ON ARRIVAL

- As soon as you can, locate and introduce yourself briefly to parents/relatives and give them your information booklet.
- Assess the child together with your medical colleague – the medical and nursing staff at the referring hospital should provide a history and update on current management.
- Liaise closely with the nurse caring for the child. The help of this nurse could be invaluable – s/he knows the child and the layout of the unit. The nurse may be keen to assist you, having participated in the management and stabilisation of the child prior to your arrival.

While carrying out your initial assessment of the child, ascertain the following:

- If the child is ventilated, what is the size, length, position and mode of securing of the ET tube
- Is the child effectively ventilated or are there problems?
- Is there a leak around the tube?
- Were there any problems during intubation?
- Has a recent arterial blood gas analysis been undertaken?
- Where are chest and other X-rays?
- Is the child cardiovascularly stable? Are the child's heart rate and blood pressure within reasonable ranges for his/her age and condition?
- If the child has had cardiac rhythm disturbances or a cardiac arrest, ascertain if a cause was found, and the treatment required to stabilise the child's condition
- Has a 12–lead ECG been performed?
- Assess the child's current perfusion – what is the capillary refill time?
- Note peripheral and central lines, their location, patency, secureness of dressings and the fluids/drugs running through them
- Check and record the dosages of drug infusions/fluids in progress, paying particular attention if the patient is a child with a suspected congenital cardiac abnormality on a prostin E_2 infusion – this drug has been known to be confused with prostacyclin, which could have serious implications and, as the dosage is calculated in nanograms, there is increased potential for error
- Note any allergies
- Note blood/specimen results that may be available

- Has a recent blood sugar level been checked?
- What is the child's urine output like? Quantity/colour/urinalysis?
- Has s/he been catheterised?
- What are the core/peripheral temperatures?
- Does the child have any rash/cuts/bruises/superficial or more serious injuries?
- Assess and document the child's neurological status, taking into consideration drugs that have been given or are in progress.

Try to gain some space to lay out the equipment you need – ask to borrow some trolleys, as these are invaluable, enabling you to lay out drugs/equipment for any procedure you need to undertake.

When you have completed all procedures required to stabilise and treat the child, prior to preparing to leave the parents will need to be updated and see their child. Check their travel arrangements – if they are very shocked/distressed, it is inadvisable for them to drive. If a friend/relative is unable to help them, involve staff at the referring hospital in making arrangements. Many teams provide maps for parents together with their information booklet, to make their journey easier. If the parents are driving, make sure they understand that under no circumstances should they attempt to follow the ambulance as it travels with blue lights at speed back to your base. If traffic is likely to be heavy or the doctor feels it is indicated for other reasons, a police escort may be required, which will need to be organised.

BEFORE TRANSFER

- Ensure all lines are secure and labelled clearly
- Have the arterial and CVP lines and transducers been attached to the child first with tape and zeroed afterwards, to ensure accurate readings when the child is moved?
- Check that any broken limbs are securely splinted, and if used, the cervical collar is correctly positioned
- Do you have copies of notes/results, including respiratory syncytial virus (RSV) status if appropriate, transfer letter and summary, X-rays, family details?

Make sure you have the following drawn up and easily accessible:

- Arrest drugs and saline flushes, all clearly labelled

- Boluses of paralysis/sedation if infusions of these are not in progress
- Volume, e.g. 4.5% albumin/blood if indicated and available (either fill and seal syringes or use a closed system through a three-way tap to avoid spillage)
- Re-intubation equipment including mask and airway, Magill's forceps, laryngoscope, ET tubes, tape, etc.
- When the child is wrapped in space blanket/gamgee/blankets and positioned on the ambulance trolley, make sure you can still gain swift access to a central/peripheral line to give drugs/fluid – cutting a square out of gamgee and a space blanket can be effective
- If you are transporting an infant, a portable incubator may be used; otherwise ensure that the infant's head is covered to conserve heat
- Consider with all children their temperature, illness, the season and length of the journey
- Suction well down the ET tube before leaving; saline may be helpful if the secretions are thick
- Consider taking additional suction catheters from the referring unit if secretions are copious and you need to add to your own supply
- Telephone base prior to leaving – update them on the condition of the child, what is needed on your return, e.g. type of ventilator/oscillator/dialysis/drug infusions, family details, accommodation requirements and their mode of travel
- Give the unit your estimated time of arrival.

IN TRANSIT

- Check that the ambulance suction is working and that the suction catheters fit the tubing (a Yankuer sucker or connector is required with some types) – some teams take their own portable suction
- Change from the portable O_2 cylinder to the ambulance supply
- Check that all your emergency equipment and drugs are nearby and not moving around the ambulance
- Check that the monitor and pumps are secure, that alarms are appropriately set and that you have a clear view of all these pieces of equipment
- Ask the crew to adjust the temperature of the ambulance according to your needs

- Some teams carry portable blood gas analysers, others find end-tidal CO_2 monitors useful in assessing the child's ventilation requirements

- If the ventilated child is going to be hand-bagged for any reason, you might be able to take turns doing this with the doctor – it can be a tiring job on a long journey!

- Make sure you use your seatbelt

- If you need to administer treatment, ask the ambulance crew to slow down/stop

- Record observations, drug dosages, etc. according to your unit policy – commonly this is done every 15 min

- Observe the child and monitors closely for signs of deterioration in vital signs/lightening level of consciousness/fitting

- In the event of an acute deterioration, the ambulance will need to pull over and stop, and you may need to request the help of the crew, for instance if the child has a cardiac arrest

- In these situations, a call ahead to your unit to inform them of a major problem will enable them to assist you immediately on arrival if required.

LOOKING AFTER YOURSELF

Retrievals can involve many hours of travelling and working in hot, stressful conditions. It is a good idea to take cartons of juice and snacks with you, and the referring unit may offer tea or coffee. Some people find nausea a problem, particularly on long journeys in the back of a swaying ambulance. Many of the new ambulances have forward-facing seats, which can help, as can opening the sliding windows a little to let some air in. Some people find sweets helpful and mints are highly recommended! If nausea becomes a real problem on retrieval journeys, you may need to consider trying 'sea bands' or appropriate medication to relieve it.

Remember to update the referring unit regularly on the condition of the child, particularly shortly after admission, and when the child leaves the unit.

Air retrievals have not been discussed here – they carry their own specific problems, whether using a fixed-wing or helicopter service, and staff need to be fully familiar with these.

REFERENCES

British Paediatric Association 1993 Report of a working party on paediatric intensive care. British Paediatric Association, London

Britto J, Nadel S, Maconochie I, Levin M, Habibi P 1995 Morbidity and severity of illness during interhospital transfer: impact of a specialist paediatric retrieval team. Br Med J 311: 836–839

Department of Health 1997a Paediatric intensive care: a framework for the future. Department of Health, London

Department of Health 1997b A bridge to the future: nursing standards, education and workforce planning in paediatric intensive care. Department of Health, London

PICS 1996 Standards for paediatric intensive care. Paediatric Intensive Care Society, London

UKCC 1992 Scope of professional practice. United Kingdom Central Council for Nursing, Health Visiting and Midwifery, London

DEATH OF A CHILD 12

THE NURSE'S ROLE

When a child dies suddenly in hospital, nurses play a central role in caring for the parents and providing essential information. Parents should be offered a private place to hold, cuddle, wash, dress or just to be near their child for as long as they wish and a nurse should be available to support the parents if desired. A telephone should be made available for their use to contact close family and friends. Often, when babies or young children die, parents like to have hand and footprints made to treasure and keep. Many parents like to keep a lock of their child's hair, but permission should be sought before taking it. A photograph is usually taken of the child when all invasive lines and medical equipment have been removed and s/he has been washed and dressed. A photograph including the family also may be helpful for the parents to keep at this time. Some parents want the photograph at the time, but a few may call after several weeks asking for it, and it must be kept safely. Often a favourite toy, a piece of jewellery, a rosary or a hand-made card from a sibling is left with the child who has died and may be buried with them. Specialist nurses, e.g. a family support sister, if in post, should be informed of each child's death and given all the relevant details and particular circumstances so that they can maintain contact with the family and provide follow-up care.

Parents should be given written information, including:

- detail of possible coroner involvement and post mortem
- when and where to collect the death certificate
- how to register the child's death
- who to contact to arrange a funeral and information regarding the Social Fund, if paying for the child's funeral may pose a problem
- addresses of support groups
- a date for the family to come back to see the consultant if they wish to discuss any unanswered issues
- the name of a known nurse who cared for the child and family whom they can contact at work if they need any other information or help.

The nurse and doctor caring for the child at the time of their death must ensure that the general practitioner, health visitor and, if appropriate, the referring hospital are informed of the child's death as soon as possible.

BRAIN STEM DEATH

The Department of Health set up a Working Party in 1998 which devised *A Code of Practice for the Diagnosis of Brain Stem Death* and their definition of death is: `irreversible loss of capacity for consciousness, combined with irreversible loss of the capacity to breathe'. Brain stem death may occur before cardiorespiratory function ceases. It is important that nurses understand and can explain the concept of brain stem death. Brain stem death tests are usually carried out by the consultant in charge of the child's care and one other clinically independent doctor, competent in the field and not a member of the transplant team, who has been qualified for at least 5 years. The tests are performed twice and, prior to testing, time must have elapsed to ensure that the patient has no circulating or therapeutic levels of any drug that could cause coma. A diagnosis must have been established and the cause of the coma must be irreversible. Prior to testing, the child should be normothermic, with no endocrine or metabolic disturbances, and have no effects of muscle relaxants in his/her system.

The British Paediatric Association (1991) guidelines for paediatric brain stem testing recommend that the child should be a minimum age of 37 weeks gestation plus 2 months, as it is rarely possible to confidently diagnose brain stem death between the ages of 37 weeks gestation and 2 months of age. Below the age of 37 weeks gestation the criteria for brainstem death cannot be applied.

Clinical tests for brain stem death

• Pupils are fixed and dilated and do not react to light.

• Absent corneal reflexes – tested by touching exposed cornea with a piece of cotton wool but taking care to avoid damage.

• Absent oculovestibular reflexes – ice cold water is syringed into each ear in turn, having ensured that the passage to the tympanic membrane is clear. Normally this would produce eye movement, where there is deviation to the stimulated side.

• No cranial nerve motor response to deep, painful stimulation within the cranial nerve distribution.

• Absent cough or gag reflex – this is tested with deep suction via the endotracheal tube and to the back of the throat.

• Apnoea test – the partial pressure of carbon dioxide (P_aCO_2) should be 5.3 kPa (40 mmHg) prior to the apnoea test and should rise to at least 6.6 kPa (50 mmHg) during the test if the patient remains apnoeic. The patient should be preoxygenated with 100% oxygen for 10 min prior to testing and arterial blood gases should be taken. The patient is disconnected from the ventilator but given a continuous supply of 100% oxygen via the endotracheal tube. The patient is observed for 10 min to note any respiratory effort and then another arterial blood gas is taken to ensure that the P_aCO_a has risen above 6.6 kPa (50 mmHg). The patient is then reconnected to the ventilator. This test must be discontinued if hypotension, cardiac arrhythmias or hypoxia occurs.

If the first test shows brain stem death, the legal time of death is recorded on completion of this first set of brain stem tests and must be declared in the medical notes. Death is not pronounced until the second set of tests has been completed.

Spinal reflexes – the spinal cord may continue to function after the death of the brain stem, and the resulting limb movement may be distressing to the family and staff caring for the patient. Nurses should be aware of this potential occurrence and be able to give the family an explanation.

If appropriate, the opportunity for organ donation must be offered to families once brain stem death has been established.

If a patient does not fulfil brain stem death criteria but has an extremely poor prognosis and a medical decision has been made to withdraw treatment, it may be possible for the patient to donate kidneys on asystole. The Transplant Co-ordinator should be contacted prior to the withdrawal of treatment to discuss the suitability of donation.

The Human Tissue Act 1961

This Act states that organ retrieval cannot be authorised (even where the wishes of the deceased are known) if: 'any surviving relative of the deceased objects to the body being so dealt with'.

THE PROCESS OF ORGAN DONATION

When a child is found to be brain stem dead, the family is offered the opportunity to donate their child's organs. The family will need time and privacy to discuss the matter and, if they are considering donation, the Transplant Co-ordinator is contacted. S/he will come to the unit to discuss all aspects with the family. If the family still wish to continue, full explanations should be given at this time about the likelihood of needing to continue treatment to maintain the organs in the best possible condition. It must be consistently reinforced that the child is brain stem dead and that no treatment can change that. Consent will then be obtained if the family wish to proceed with the donation of their child's organs.

Once recipients have been found for the organs, a team of doctors will usually come to retrieve the organs. Major organs will not be removed unless a matched recipient has been identified. The donor's family will usually say their goodbyes at this time, then the child is taken to theatre with cardiopulmonary function being maintained and supported.

Once the organs have been retrieved, they are taken, swiftly, to be transplanted into the recipients. The donor child's body will be carefully sutured and then taken to the mortuary or back to the ward if the parents wish to spend more time saying their goodbyes. The time taken between parents deciding to donate their child's organs and the time the child is actually taken to theatre is usually 12–24 hours, and parents have the right to change their mind at any time. The process described is concerned with large organ donation, as some tissues, e.g. heart valves and corneas, may be retrieved the following day.

NB The parents may wish to come back to see their child in the hospital chapel following donation of their child's organs, and they may wish to hold and cuddle their child, so it may be advisable to gently inform them that:

- their child will feel cold to the touch
- their child will look very pale
- their child will have a suture line where the organs have been removed
- their child may feel lighter in weight if they pick him/her up for a cuddle
- their child's abdomen may appear concave if large organs have been donated.

MULTIORGAN DONATION

Age criteria

- *Kidneys*: 2–75 years (paediatric donors are assessed according to size and weight)
- *Liver*: 0–70 years
- *Heart*: 0–60 years (if unsuitable, the heart valves may be considered)
- *Lungs*: 0–60 years
- *Pancreas*: 18–45 years (outside these age limits, the pancreas may be donated for research).

Other criteria

- Age, as previously described, according to the British Paediatric Association guidelines
- A confirmed diagnosis of brain stem death
- Artificially ventilated
- No past medical or social history contraindications – no current or past history of malignancy, except for tissue-diagnosed primary brain tumour and not categorised high-risk
- Coroner's consent
- Consent from legal next of kin
- Virology screen (negative HIV and Hepatitis B and C).

Multiorgan donors may also donate tissues

- *Corneas*: 6 months–100 years (poor eyesight is not a contraindication)
- *Heart valves*: 6 months–60 years.

(Trachea and skin may also be donated, but not from paediatric patients.)

Investigations that may be required prior to organ donation

This is the responsibility of the transplant co-ordinator but it requires team work and it may be helpful to liaise with the co-ordinator and to begin to obtain the necessary tests so that the process takes as little time as possible.

- Virology screen – 10 mL of blood in plain blood tube (it may be necessary to take a virology screen from the mother if the child is under 2 years of age)
- Blood group
- Urea and electrolytes
- Liver function tests
- Arterial blood gases
- Clotting studies
- Sputum Gram stain
- Chest X-ray
- ECG
- Amylase
- Echocardiogram
- Culture and sensitivity screens – wounds, sputum, urine.

CLINICAL MANAGEMENT GUIDELINES OF THE ORGAN DONOR

(Reproduced with permission from Marchant 1997.)

Common clinical problems that may occur in a brain stem dead patient include:

- Hypotension
- Hypothermia
- Endocrine disturbances
- Electrolyte imbalance
- Arrhythmias
- Hypoxia
- Coagulopathy
- Neurogenic pulmonary oedema.

Hypotension

Causes: Loss of vasomotor tone, myocardial depression, hypovolaemia due to blood loss, diuretics, vasodilation or diabetes insipidus.

Effect: Poor organ perfusion with potential ischaemia.

Management: Filling, preferably with colloid solution, inotropes – dobutamine, dopamine and epinephrine – as a last resort.

Goal: Normotension, CVP 5–10 cmH$_2$O, urine output 1 mL./kg/min.

Hypothermia

Causes: Loss of temperature regulation and vasomotor tone aggravated by hypovolaemia.

Effect: Risk of arrhythmias, decreased basal metabolic rate, increased oxidisers.

Management: Warm slowly using warming blanket, warm IV fluids, warm inhaled gases.

Goal: Temperature 35–37°C.

Endocrine disturbances – diabetes insipidus

Causes: Cerebral ischaemia, raised intracranial pressure, hypoxia.

Effect: Polyuria causing gross hypovolaemia, electrolyte imbalance.

Management: Do not fluid deplete, DO NOT STOP DOPAMINE, investigate fluid replacement therapy, administer DDAVP but avoid giving this within 2 h of going to theatre.

Goal: Normalise urine output and concentration.

Electrolyte imbalance

Common electrolyte disturbances experienced are hypokalaemia, hypocalcaemia and hypernatraemia.

Causes: Blood loss, diabetes insipidus, inadequate replacement therapy.

Effect: Cardiac arrhythmia, poor cardiac contractility, asystole.

Management: Monitor and correct imbalance.

Goal: Normal values.

Hypoxia

Causes: Trauma, aspiration, sputum retention, pulmonary oedema.

Effect: Poor tissue and organ perfusion.

Management: Physiotherapy, including bagging and suction, frequent turning, bronchoscopy, correct CO_2 and frequent ABG, avoid excessive crystalloid infusion, add PEEP.

Goal: P_aO_2 >11.0 kPa (>83 mmHg), airway pressures <30 cmH$_2$O, clear chest X-ray, F$_i$O$_2$ <0.4, audible clear air entry.

Coagulopathy

Causes: The ischaemic brain and resultant catecholamine storm releases fibrinolytic agents into the circulation.

Effect: Presentation of a DIC-type picture.

Management: Administration of relevant clotting factors, monitor clotting studies, observe for clinical signs of haemorrhage, rule out possibility of underlying, undiagnosed haematological disorder.

Neurogenic pulmonary oedema

Causes: Catecholamine surge in response to intracranial insult may cause a sudden increase in systemic vascular resistance, with a shift of blood flow from the systemic circulation to the pulmonary circulation.

Effect: Hypoxia leading to poor tissue and organ perfusion.

Management: Assess fluid status, redo chest X-ray, consider reversing I:E ratio, add PEEP, continue to monitor blood gases, continue physiotherapy, DO NOT GIVE UP.

Goal: Normalised arterial blood gases with no pulmonary oedema. If management is unsuccessful, the lungs may be unsuitable for donation.

 Discuss the necessity to continue all medication with the Transplant Co-ordinator (if antibiotics are stopped too soon, transplant teams may reject the organs of a septic patient).

RELIGION

There are no religious denominations that object to organ or tissue donation; however, it is advisable to be aware of individual requirements for the care of the deceased. It may be important for the next of kin to liaise with their religious leader regarding donation. This is always respected.

REFERENCES

Conference of Medical Royal Colleges and their Faculties in the United Kingdom 1991 Diagnosis of brainstem death in infants and children. British Paediatric Association, London

Department of Health 1998 A code of practice for the diagnosis of brain stem death: including guidelines for the identification and management of potential organ and tissue donors. HMSO, London

Human Tissue Act 1961 HMSO, London

Marchant C 1997 The organ donation information folder. South Thames Transplant Co-ordination Service, London

13

It is useful for nurses to have some knowledge of normal child development in order to be able to assess a child thoroughly on admission. Each child is different and the parents/carers may be the best source of information about developmental milestones achieved. It has been shown that some children regress developmentally when they are admitted to hospital or in other stressful circumstances. This chapter is intended as a guide to normal child development. Growth assessment (centile) charts are included to plot the child's length, weight and head circumference at the end of the chapter. These can be used as an initial assessment tool but are most useful when data is plotted over time.

STAGES OF COGNITIVE DEVELOPMENT (PIAGET & INHELDER 1969)

- 0–2 years – sensorimotor stage
- 2–6 years – preoperational stage
- 6–12 years – concrete operational stage
- 12 years+ – formal operational stage.

Sensorimotor stage

The infant's response to the world is almost entirely sensory and motor. This stage may be subdivided into six substages:

- 0–1 month – reflexes
- 1–4 months – primary circular reactions (e.g. putting finger into mouth)
- 4–10 months – secondary circular reactions (i.e. beginning to realise that own actions have external results)
- 10 months – 1 year – co-ordination of secondary schemes (i.e. combining actions to achieve a result)
- 1–1.5 years – tertiary circular actions (improving motor skills)
- 1.5–2 years – beginning of thought.

Box 13.1 Seven major reflexes in the newborn (from Bee 1989)

- Rooting – infant will turn towards the touch of a cheek, searching for something to suck
- Sucking – sucking results from putting something into the infant's mouth
- Swallowing – initially not well co-ordinated with breathing
- Moro – when startled, infants will arch their back and throw open their arms
- Grasp – infants will curl their fingers around any object that can be grasped
- Babinski – if an infant is stroked on the bottom of the foot, the toes splay out, then curl in
- Stepping – if infants are held so that their feet just touch the ground, they will initiate walking movements

---

Preoperational stage

This stage involves the use of images, words or actions that convey something else, e.g. pretend play. Initially children in this stage are egocentric – they see the world only in their own perspective – but this view widens during this stage as the child learns to share.

Concrete operational stage

During this stage logic and reasoning develop. The child begins to understand the concept of reversibility and the principles of conservation.

Formal operational stage

During this stage the child develops deductive reasoning and a systematic problem-solving approach.

FREUD'S STAGES OF PSYCHOSEXUAL DEVELOPMENT

Freud (1964) looked differently at child development, as shown in Table 13.1.

Table 13.1	Freud's stages of psychosexual development	
Age	**Stage**	**Developmental task**
0–1 year	Oral	Weaning
2–3 years	Anal	Toilet training
4–5 years	Phallic	Identification with parent of same sex
6–12 years	Latency	Development of ego
13–18 years	Genital	Mature sexual intimacy

NORMAL CHILD DEVELOPMENT – WHAT TO EXPECT OF A CHILD OF A CERTAIN AGE (WHALEY & WONG 1991, ENGEL 1993)

Newborn

- Reflexes as previously described
- Normal range of cries, including differing cries for hunger or pain
- Vision: best able to focus eyes at a distance of 25 cm
- Unable to hold head up but can turn head to side when prone
- Hands held with fingers curled into a fist.

Six weeks

- Starts to smile
- Starts to coo in response to the sound of mother's voice
- Developing head control.

Three months

- Starts laughing
- Can hold head up beyond the plane of the rest of the body
- Has only slight head lag when pulled to sit
- Follows an object for 180° when lying supine
- Turns head to sound
- Posterior fontanelle now closed.

Six months

- No head lag when pulled to sit
- Sits without support

- Starts babbling
- Teething begins
- Can chew on soft food
- Can transfer object from one hand to another
- Increasing fear of strangers.

Nine months

- Pulls to a standing position
- Crawls on tummy
- Babbles repetitive syllables
- Can pick up a small object between thumb and forefinger.

One year

- Walks with one hand held
- Knows own name
- Can speak 2–3 words clearly
- Can drink from cup with help
- Begins casting objects
- Clings to mother when in unfamiliar situations.

Eighteen months

- Begins to identify objects
- Vocabulary around 50 words
- Begins to combine two words as a sentence
- Points to object and can feed self
- Jumps using both feet
- Can build a tower of 3–4 cubes
- Begins to scribble
- Anterior fontanelle closes
- Can use a spoon but will turn it upside down before it reaches the mouth.

Two years

- Talks to self during play
- Vocabulary around 300 words
- Knows 4 body parts
- Can put on pants, socks and shoes
- Mainly dry at night.

Four years

- Has conversational speech
- Can write own name
- Can count
- Vocabulary of around 1500 words
- Can dress and undress
- Enjoys imaginary play.

Six years

- Vocabulary of several thousand words
- Increasing dexterity, can run, jump and ride a bike
- Knows right from left
- May show jealousy of siblings
- Enjoys playing games.

Eight years

- Increasing manual dexterity, can use most household utensils
- Learns principles of conversation
- Keen to be involved in clubs, likes company of others
- Able to classify
- Can count backwards from 20
- Likes to help.

Ten years

- Height slowly increasing
- Weight increasing rapidly
- Start of puberty for some children
- Has logical thinking
- Best friends are important
- Can wash and dry own hair
- May begin to show interest in the opposite sex.

Adolescence

- Increasing weight and height
- Girls may commence menstruation
- Bodily changes associated with puberty
- Mood swings
- Conflicts with parents
- Increasing capacity for abstract reasoning
- Developing sexual identity.

CHILDREN'S DEVELOPMENTAL CONCEPTS OF PAIN

It is important that nurses understand children's cognitive development and their perceptions of pain at each developmental stage.

Hurley & Whelan (1988) describe children's concepts of pain according to Piaget's cognitive developmental stages. The sensorimotor stage is omitted as these children are unable to vocalise their perceptions of pain.

Preoperational stage (2–7 years)

- These children may think that pain is a punishment for something that they have done wrong
- They may blame someone else for their pain
- They relate to pain primarily as a physical experience
- They often have feelings of sadness when in pain so may feel comforted if held and given reassurance.

Concrete operational stage (7–10 years)

- These children can understand physical pain and can locate the pain to the relevant part of the body
- They fear bodily harm and death
- They like to feel they have some control over the pain so they should be encouraged to ask for help to find the most comfortable position or to ask for pain relief.

Formal operational stage (12 years +)

- These children are able to use reasoning, e.g. my head hurts because I banged it.
- They fear loss of privacy and control when in pain
- They need to be given as much information as they require and choices about how best to control the pain.

GROWTH ASSESSMENT CHARTS FOR BOYS AND GIRLS
(BUCKLER & TANNER 1995)

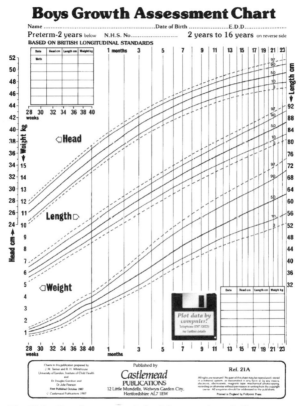

Fig. 13.1 Growth assessment chart: boys, preterm to 2 years (reproduced with permission of Castelmead Publications, Welwyn Garden City)

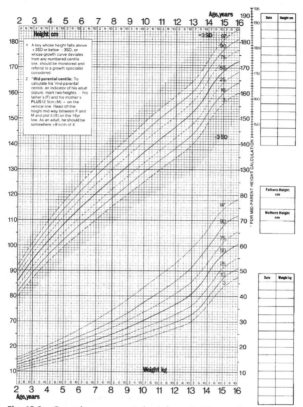

Fig. 13.2 Growth assessment chart: boys, 2–16 years (reproduced with permission of Castelmead Publications, Welwyn Garden City)

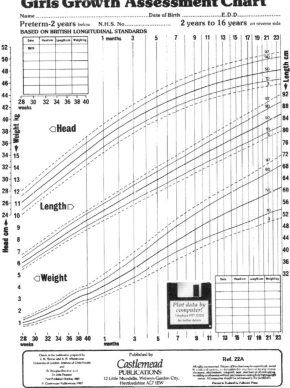

Fig. 13.3 Growth assessment chart: girls, preterm to 2 years (reproduced with permission of Castelmead Publications, Welwyn Garden City)

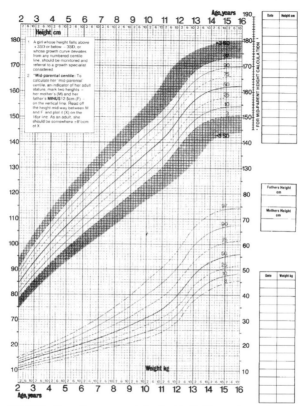

Fig. 13.4 Growth assessment chart: girls, 2–16 years (reproduced with permission of Castelmead Publications, Welwyn Garden City)

REFERENCES

Bee H 1989 The developing child, 5th edn. Harper & Row, New York

Buckler J M H, Tanner J M 1995 Girls and boys height and weight charts. Castlemead Publications, Welwyn Garden City, Herts

Engel J 1993 Pocket guide pediatric assessment, 2nd edn. C V Mosby, St Louis, MO

Freud S 1964 An outline of psychoanalysis. Hogarth Press, London

Hurley A, Whelan E G 1988 Cognitive development and children's perception of pain. Pediat Nurs 14(1): 21–24

Piaget J, Inhelder B 1969 The psychology of the child. Routledge & Kegan Paul, London

Whaley L F, Wong D L 1991 Nursing care of infants and children, 4th edn. C V Mosby, St Louis, MO

FURTHER READING

Illingworth R S 1993 The normal child, 10th edn. Churchill Livingstone, Edinburgh

Sylva K, Lunt I 1990 Child development: a first course. Blackwell, Oxford

QUICK REFERENCE TO SYNDROMES

Infants and children may present in Accident and Emergency or a PICU with a collection of unexplained symptoms and signs that may lead to diagnosis of a previously undiagnosed syndrome. The following list is not comprehensive but provides a quick reference to the more common syndromes.

The term 'congenital' means existing at and usually before birth.

CHROMOSOMAL DISORDERS

There may be addition or deletion of chromosomes.

Cri du chat syndrome

This syndrome occurs as a result of partial deletion of the short arm of chromosome 5. A characteristic of this syndrome is a high-pitched cry, which resembles the 'cry' of a cat.

Appearance: Craniofacial abnormalities, microcephaly and a moon-shaped face with hypertelorism (increased interpupillary distance).

These children have severe learning difficulties and an increased incidence of congenital heart defects.

DiGeorge syndrome

This syndrome is usually a sporadic malformation but some patients show a microdeletion of chromosome 22. The thymus and parathyroid glands are absent because of defective development of the third and fourth embryonic pharyngeal pouches. This is characterised by neonatal tetany, hypocalcaemia and frequent viral infections.

Appearance: dysmorphic features.
There may be aortic arch anomalies.

Down syndrome (trisomy 21)

An extra chromosome 21 characterises the best recognised of chromosome disorders.

Appearance: Small, slanting eyes, low-set ears, prominent epicanthic (neck) folds, small mouth causing frequent tongue protrusion and commonly there is a single transverse palmar crease.

These children will have learning difficulties with a reduced IQ. Down syndrome is often associated with a congenital heart lesion, umbilical hernia, higher than normal incidence of duodenal atresia, Hirschsprung's disease and leukaemia.

Edward syndrome (trisomy 18)

Appearance: The baby will have protruding eyes, low-set malformed ears, a receding chin, flexion deformities of the hands with the index finger overlapping the third digit, and characteristic feet with a prominent heel and convex sole ('rocker-bottom feet'). Infants usually have major cardiac anomalies and survival is uncommon beyond six months.

Klinefelter syndrome (XXY)

This syndrome affects males only and means that their chromosome pattern is XXY and they are infertile. It is often undiagnosed until adolescence.

Appearance: Tall in stature with unusually long legs, hypogonadism and gynaecomastia. There is increased incidence of learning difficulties.

Prader–Willi syndrome

In approximately 50% of patients with this syndrome there is a small deletion in the long arm on chromosome 15 (Connor & Ferguson-Smith 1987).

Appearance: Round face with a prominent forehead and a pronounced nasal bridge, short stature, small hands and feet, obesity and hypogonadism.

These children are initially hypotonic and have delayed motor development, feeding difficulties and learning difficulties.

Turner syndrome (X)

This syndrome affects females only. They have only 45 chromosomes and have a chromosome pattern of XO.

Appearance: Short stature, micrognathia (small jaw), webbing of the neck, lymphoedema, widely-spaced nipples, failure to develop breasts.

Normal lifespan and intelligence, but increased incidence of congenital heart defects, particularly coarctation of the aorta and atrial septal defect. Most females with Turner syndrome are infertile.

MUCOPOLYSACCHARIDOSES

There are four main types:

Type 1 – Hurler syndrome

This is a sex linked recessive trait that affects only males. It results from a deficiency of the enzyme α-L-iduronidase.

Appearance: Abnormal facial features, an enlarged tongue, clouded corneas, short neck and trunk, joint deformities and angular kyphosis.

Hepatosplenomegaly, deafness and cardiac defects are common and the children will have learning difficulties. Large quantities of dermatan sulphate are present in the urine.

Type 2 – Hunter syndrome

This syndrome is also an autosomal recessive trait that affects only males. The symptoms in Hunter syndrome are generally milder than those in Hurler syndrome.

Appearance: Some facial abnormalities but in a milder form than in type 1, angular kyphosis, nodular skin lesions but generally no clouding of the corneas.

These children may also have retinitis pigmentosa, optic atrophy, progressive deafness and pulmonary hypertension. Large quantities of dermatan or heparin sulphate may be present in the urine.

Type 3 – Sanfilippo syndrome

This syndrome has autosomal recessive inheritance. There is a deficiency of either heparin sulphate sulphamidase or N-acetyl-α-D-glucosaminidase. These children have severe progressive learning difficulties but normal features, no corneal clouding and no cardiac defects.

Type 4 – Morquio syndrome

This is a rare form of mucopolysaccharidosis that again is an autosomal recessive trait.

Appearance: Short stature, short neck, prominent sternum, scoliosis, waddling gait, protruding mandible and short nose.

These children have normal intelligence but may have mild deafness, clouding of the cornea and perhaps aortic valve disease.

CONGENITAL MALFORMATIONS AND DYSMORPHIC SYNDROMES

The CHARGE and VATER association of symptoms are included in this section.

CHARGE association

CHARGE is an acronym of congenital defects that can occur together:

C Coloboma – this is a malformation that results in a cleft in one of the structures of the eye, most commonly the iris
H Heart defects
A choanal Atresia
R Retarded growth and development
G Genital hypoplasia
E Ear anomalies/deafness.

Children with CHARGE association may also have renal anomalies, tracheo-oesophageal fistula and orofacial problems (Contact-a-Family 1996).

Noonan syndrome

This is an autosomal dominant trait that affects both sexes but is sometimes known as male Turner syndrome.

Appearance: Downwards slanting eyes, low-set ears, webbed neck and short stature.

Learning difficulties and congenital heart defects (most commonly hypertrophic cardiomyopathy or pulmonary stenosis) are often present.

Pierre Robin syndrome

In this syndrome there is underdevelopment of the lower jaw, micrognathia and glossoptosis (downwards displacement of the tongue), often associated with cleft palate and absent gag reflex. Infants should be nursed on their sides or prone as the tongue is at risk of occluding the airway.

Sturge–Weber syndrome

This is a congenital syndrome that affects the brain, skin and eyes.

Appearance: Facial haemangioma (port-wine stain).

Intracranial haemangioma is associated with the facial haemangioma. Focal seizures, learning difficulties and glaucoma may occur.

Treacher Collins syndrome (mandibulofacial dysostosis)

This is an autosomal dominant trait.

Appearance: Characteristic facial appearance – sloping downwards eyes, flat cheeks, hypoplastic mandible, receding chin, large mouth, high palate, low-set ears and deficient cartilage, sometimes with no auditory meatus.

VATER association

This is an acronym for a combination of malformations:

V Vertebral defects
A Anal atresia
TE Tracheo-oEsophageal fistula
R Renal defects, radial limb dysplasia.

These children have normal intelligence but may also have congenital heart disease.

Wolff–Parkinson–White syndrome

This is a tachydysrhythmia. Cardiac electrical impulses are transmitted along an accessory pathway and therefore atrial impulses can bypass the normal delay that usually occurs at the atrioventricular node. This leads to a rapid re-entry SVT and a characteristic ECG trace with a short P–R interval and a wide QRS interval.

REFERENCES

Connor J M, Ferguson-Smith M A 1987 Essential medical genetics, 2nd edn. Blackwell, Oxford

Contact-a-Family 1996 Directory of specific conditions and rare syndromes in children and their family support networks, 3rd edn. Contact-a-Family, London

---

FURTHER READING

Hull D, Johnston D I 1985 Essential paediatrics. Churchill Livingstone, Edinburgh

Jolly H, Levene M I 1985 Diseases of children, 5th edn. Blackwell, Oxford

Whaley L F, Wong D L 1991 Nursing care of infants and children, 4th edn. C V Mosby, St Louis, MO

INDEX